THE COVID-19 PANDEMIC AND THE POLITICS OF LIFE

This book explores the extent to which the COVID-19 pandemic is poised to be a permanent fixture in the modern world which in contemporary times will be thought of in terms of before and after the pandemic. It looks at how the pandemic has brought to the fore the question of the appropriate ethics, politics, and spirituality and highlights the present condition of humanity and the need to rethink alternative planetary futures. It argues that the pandemic has existential and epistemic implications for human life on planet Earth, and a post–COVID-19 future requires a fundamental transformation of the present economic, political, and social conditions.

Drawing on empirical case studies on the COVID-19 pandemic from Africa and beyond, contributions in this book challenge the reader to rethink alternative planetary futures. It will be a useful resource for students, scholars, and researchers of African studies, citizenship studies, global development, global politics, human geography, migration studies, development studies, international studies, international relations, and political science.

Inocent Moyo is an Associate Professor in the Department of Geography and Environmental Studies and Acting Deputy Dean of Research, Innovation, and Internationalisation in the Faculty of Science, Agriculture, and Engineering at the University of Zululand, South Africa. He researches borders, migration, and the political economy of the informal economy in the Southern African region.

Sabelo J. Ndlovu-Gatsheni is Research Chair in Epistemologies of the Global South at the University of Bayreuth, Germany. He is a prominent historian and one of the leading decolonial scholars and theorists in the Global South. He was the Executive Director of the Change Management Unit (CMU) in the Principal and Vice-Chancellor's office at the University of South Africa (UNISA) and Professor of African Political Economy at the Thabo Mbeki African Leadership Institute (TMALI) at the same institution. Previously, he headed the Archie Mafeje Research Institute for Applied Social Policy (AMRI).

THE COVID-19 PANDEMIC AND THE POLITICS OF LIFE

Edited by Inocent Moyo
and Sabelo J. Ndlovu-Gatsheni

Routledge
Taylor & Francis Group

LONDON AND NEW YORK

Designed cover image: © Getty Images / AdrianHillman

First published 2024
by Routledge
4 Park Square, Milton Park, Abingdon, Oxon OX14 4RN

and by Routledge
605 Third Avenue, New York, NY 10158

Routledge is an imprint of the Taylor & Francis Group, an informa business

British Library Cataloguing-in-Publication Data
A catalogue record for this book is available from the British Library

Library of Congress Cataloging-in-Publication Data
Names: Moyo, Inocent, editor. | Ndlovu-Gatsheni, Sabelo J., editor.
Title: The COVID-19 pandemic and the politics of life / edited by Inocent
  Moyo, Sabelo J. Ndlovu-Gatsheni.
Description: Abingdon, Oxon ; New York, NY : Routledge, 2024. | Includes bibliographical
  references and index.
Summary: "This book explores the extent to which the COVID-19 pandemic is poised to
  be a permanent temporality in the modern world in which contemporary time will be
  thought of in terms of before and after the pandemic. It looks at how the pandemic
  has brought to the fore the question of appropriate ethics, politics, and spirituality and highlights
  the present condition of humanity and the need to rethink alternative planetary futures. It argues
  that the pandemic has existential and epistemic implications for human life on planet earth and
  post-COVID-19 futures require a fundamental transformation of the present economic, political,
  and social conditions. Drawing on empirical case studies on the COVID-19 pandemic from
  Africa and beyond, contributions in this book challenge the reader to rethink alternative
  planetary futures. It will be a useful resource for students, scholars, and researchers of African
  studies, citizenship studies, global development, global politics, human geography, migration
  studies, development studies, international studies, international relations, and political
  science"— Provided by publisher.
Identifiers: LCCN 2023005085 (print) | LCCN 2023005086 (ebook) |
  ISBN 9781032404509 (hardback) | ISBN 9781032540993 (paperback) |
  ISBN 9781003415121 (ebook)
Subjects: LCSH: COVID-19 Pandemic, 2020—Political aspects—Case
  studies. | COVID-19 Pandemic, 2020—Social aspects—Case studies.
Classification: LCC RA644.C67 C6884 2024 (print) | LCC RA644.C67
  (ebook) | DDC 616.2/4144—dc23/eng/20230407
LC record available at https://lccn.loc.gov/2023005085
LC ebook record available at https://lccn.loc.gov/2023005086

ISBN: 978-1-032-40450-9 (hbk)
ISBN: 978-1-032-54099-3 (pbk)
ISBN: 978-1-003-41512-1 (ebk)

DOI: 10.4324/9781003415121

Typeset in Bembo
by Apex CoVantage, LLC

CONTENTS

Notes on Contributors   *vii*

1 The planetary impact of COVID-19   1
   Inocent Moyo and Sabelo J. Ndlovu-Gatsheni

2 Reengaging power: state responses to COVID-19 and the
   provision of public goods in Canada and the United States
   of America   9
   Samuel Ojo Oloruntoba and Kgoto Jan Mbele

3 COVID-19 and the challenges of trauma, transformations,
   and deborderisation: ethics, politics, and spirituality and
   alternative planetary futures   29
   Ananta Kumar Giri

4 The COVID-19 moment: exacerbation of narrow
   nationalisms and their toxicity to integration aspirations   42
   Zenzo Moyo

5 COVID-19 pandemic, geopolitics of health, and security
   entanglement in West Africa   60
   Olukayode A. Faleye

6 The conundrum of balancing between COVID-19 policing and human rights protection in South Africa: a responsibility to protect perspective (R2P) 75
Patrick Dzimiri

7 A Trojan horse: critically exploring data as a colonial instrument during the COVID-19 pandemic in South Africa 90
Kyle John Bester and Danille Elize Arendse

8 Occupational health in the mining industry of South Africa and the COVID-19 pandemic 109
Robert Maseko

9 "On est pas de cobayes": Congolese migrants and health transnationalism in the COVID-19 moment 127
Leon Mwamba Tshimpaka and Christopher Changwe Nshimbi

10 "#Corona Jihad": remanufacturing Islamophobic narratives during COVID-19 in contemporary India 141
Sayan Dey

Index 160

NOTES ON CONTRIBUTORS

Danille Elize Arendse obtained a BA (psychology), BA Honours degree (Psychology) and MA (Research Psychology) degree from the University of the Western Cape. She joined the SANDF in 2011 as a uniformed member and became employed as a Research Psychologist at the Military Psychological Institute (MPI). She completed her PhD in Psychology at the University of Pretoria in 2018. She holds a Major rank and was the Research Psychology Intern Supervisor and Coordinator at MPI. She is also a Research Associate for the Department of Psychology at the University of Pretoria and an Accredited Conflict Dynamics Mediator. In 2022, she was awarded the Diverse Black Africa research grant and travel grant that is affiliated with Michigan State University. She is currently a postdoctoral fellow at the Centre for the Study of the Afterlife of Violence and the Reparative Quest at Stellenbosch University. She is also currently funded under the NIHSS/SU prestigious postdoctoral fellowship. She has presented and published papers both locally and internationally. Her research interests include 'Coloured' identity, mentoring, psychometric assessments, cognitive psychology, psycholinguistics, military, wellbeing, gender and sexuality and decolonial research.

Kyle John Bester is a registered Research Psychologist and Cybersecurity Awareness specialist. He obtained a B.Psych (Counselling psychology) degree at Pearson Institute of Higher Education formerly known as Midrand Graduate institute in 2015. He also obtained a M.A Psychology (Masters in Research Psychology) degree from the University of the Western Cape in 2017. He joined the University of South Africa as a lecturer in psychology in 2019 and specialises in cybersecurity awareness in the South African armed forces context. He completed his PhD in Military Science at Stellenbosch University in 2023 and focused on exploring the perceptions of cybersecurity among South African military officers. He has presented and published book-chapters both locally and internationally. His research interests include military science; data-colonialism; cybersecurity awareness; Securitisation of cyber-space; Cyber-psychology.

Sayan Dey is currently working as a postdoctoral fellow at the Wits Centre for Diversity Studies, University of Witwatersrand, South Africa. He is also a faculty fellow of the Harriet Tubman Institute, York University, Canada. Some of his published books are *The Indigenous Voice of Poetomachia: The Various Perspectives of Text and Performance* (2018), *Different Spaces, Different Voices: A Rendezvous with Decoloniality* (2019), *Decolonial Existence and Urban Sensibility: A Study of Mahesh Elkunchwar* (2019), *History and Myth: Postcolonial Dimensions* (2020), *Myths, Histories and Decolonial Interventions: A Planetary Resistance* (2022), and *Green Academia: Towards Eco-friendly Education Systems* (2022). His areas of research interest are postcolonial studies, decolonial studies, critical race studies, food humanities, and critical diversity literacy.

Patrick Dzimiri is a senior lecturer and former head of department for the Department of Arts and Social Sciences, Faculty of Humanities, Social Sciences and Education, at the University of Venda. He has published in peer-reviewed journals and read papers at both international and national conferences. Having researched broadly on issues relating to global politics, governance, human rights, human security, and humanitarian affairs, of late, his research focus has slowly shifted more towards community-specific investigations, with the target of yielding tangible society and people-oriented research outcomes in areas of migration politics, electoral politics, and development politics as well as uncovering issues of inequalities in multi-cultural, multi-racial, and multi-ethnic social settings. His research focus resonates with goal 16 of the United Nations Sustainable Development Goals, which aims to promote peaceful and inclusive societies for sustainable development.

Olukayode A. Faleye is Associate Professor in history and international studies at Edo State University, Uzairue, Nigeria.

Ananta Kumar Giri is a professor at the Madras Institute of Development Studies, Chennai, India. He has been a visiting professor and researcher at many universities in India and abroad, including Aalborg University (Denmark), Maison des sciences de l'homme, Paris (France), the University of Kentucky (USA), University of Freiburg and Humboldt University (Germany), Jagiellonian University (Poland), and Jawaharlal Nehru University, New Delhi. He has an abiding interest in social movements and cultural change, criticism, creativity, and contemporary dialectics of philosophy and literature. He has written and edited around two dozen books in Odia and English, including *Social Theory and Asian Dialogues: Cultivating Planetary Conversations* (editor, 2018); *Practical Spirituality and Human Development:*

Transformations in Religions and Societies (editor, 2018); *Practical Spirituality and Human Development: Alternative Experiments for Creative Futures* (editor, 2019); and *Transformative Harmony* (editor, 2019).

Robert Maseko is a postdoctoral research Fellow at the Department of Development Studies, University of South Africa. He researches on the social condition of Black mineworkers in South Africa and labour-related studies in the Platinum Belt of South Africa. His other research interests also include issues of decoloniality, decolonisation, and colonialism.

Kgoto Jan Mbele is a PhD candidate and lecturer in the Department of Development Studies, University of South Africa. His research interests are in civil society organisations and development in Africa.

Zenzo Moyo is a scholar, researcher, and independent consultant based in the United Kingdom. He is also a research fellow at the University of Johannesburg's Department of Anthropology and Development Studies. He completed his MA (2013) and PhD (2018) in development studies at the University of Johannesburg, South Africa. His PhD thesis was on state–civil society relations and how these relations have moderated processes of democratization in Zimbabwe. His research interests are in civil society; social movements; democracy; African and opposition politics; human rights; and the interlinkages between poverty, education, and development.

Christopher Changwe Nshimbi is SARChI (South African Research Chairs Initiative) Research Chair in the Political Economy of Migration in the SADC Region and director of the Center for the Study of Governance Innovation (GovInn). He is also an associate professor in the Department of Political Sciences at the University of Pretoria, South Africa. His research focuses on migration, borders, regional integration, the informal economy, and water governance. He sits in on regional and international technical working groups on trade, labour, migration, and water governance. He is also a member of the Platform for African European Studies (PAES).

Samuel Ojo Oloruntoba is an adjunct research professor at the Institute of African Studies, Carleton University, Ottawa, Ontario, Canada, and honorary professor at the Thabo Mbeki School of Public and International Affairs, University of South Africa, where he was previously an associate professor. He obtained a PhD in political science from the University of Lagos, Nigeria. He was previously a visiting scholar at the Program of African Studies, Northwestern University, Evanston, and a fellow of Brown International Advanced Research Institute, Brown University, Rhode Island, United States of America. He is the author, editor, and co-editor of several books including *Regionalism and Integration in Africa, EU-ACP Economic Partnership Agreements and Euro-Nigeria Relations* (2016) and co-editor with Toyin Falola of the *Palgrave Handbook of Africa and the Changing Global Orde*, 2022, among others. His research interests are in the political economy of development in Africa, regional integration, migration, democracy and development, global governance of trade and finance, politics of natural resources governance and EU-African relations. He has won several awards and grants from local and international research institutions. He is also a member of the African Knowledge Network, Office of Special Adviser on Africa UN Under Secretary-General, United Nations, New York.

Leon Mwamba Tshimpaka is a postdoctoral research fellow in the Centre for the Study for Governance Innovation, SARChI Chair in the Political Economy of Migration in the SADC region, Department of Political Sciences at the University of Pretoria, and visiting scholar in the Migration and Inclusive Societies Fellowship at the University of Luxembourg. He is also an adjunct professor in the School of Liberal Arts and Humanities at Woxsen University, India, and a visiting scholar at Ku Leuven, Belgium. Dr. Tshimpaka's research includes regional integration in SADC and BRICS, EU-Africa relations, migration, political transnationalism of African migrants, civil society and consolidation of democracy in Africa, anti-corruption initiatives, and sustainable development in Africa. He obtained a PhD in political science from the University of Pretoria, South Africa, and an MA in development studies from the University of South Africa. Dr. Tshimpaka is a co-author of Regional Economic Communities and Integration in Southern Africa: Networks of Civil Society Organizations and Alternative Regionalism, published by Springer Nature in 2021, as well as the author of book chapters and journal articles. He is also an expert on European studies and a member of the Platform for African European Studies (PAES).

1

THE PLANETARY IMPACT OF COVID-19

Inocent Moyo and Sabelo J. Ndlovu-Gatsheni

Introduction

It seems that the COVID-19 pandemic is poised to be a permanent temporality in the modern world which in contemporary times will be thought of in terms of "before COVID-19" and "after COVID-19". While the "after COVID-19" is still speculation, the "before COVID-19" as a timescale is upon the modern world. This will be one of its most important abstract planetary impacts. But it has other existential and epistemic implications for human life on planet Earth as well as economic and other impacts (see Ndlovu-Gatsheni, 2020). Human health is a key existential issue. Pandemics threaten human life itself. The emergence of coronavirus and the outbreak of COVID-19 put human life on Earth at risk across the planet. The initial responses by the former president of the United States, Donald Trump, of trying to "ethnicize" the coronavirus as a "Chinese virus" (see e.g. Reja, 2021; Viala-Gaudefroy & Lindaman, 2020) did not help as the whole world was fast caught up by the COVID-19 pandemic.

Ironically, across the world a pandemic provoked national and then transnational responses. Both developed and developing countries in the wake of the COVID-19 pandemic invoked travel bans. The distinctive example is how in the period from November to December 2021, many Western European and North American countries introduced travel bans against South Africa and other southern African nation-states in response to the new COVID-19 variant, omicron. What motivated the travel bans is that in line with the World Health Organization (WHO) protocols, South Africa reported the new COVID-19 variant. The media in developed countries went into a frenzy, and this culminated in the new variant being referred to as the South African one, leading to travel bans. What is disturbing is that this new variant had been discovered in some European countries such as the Netherlands, who

DOI: 10.4324/9781003415121-1

never reported it and were never vilified, but it was huge news when South Africa made the report and thus attracted the said travel bans. It was such responses that led to the emergence of notions of COVID-colonialism capturing the attitude towards and treatment of developing countries in the response towards the COVID-19 pandemic (see e.g. Marwala, 2021; Ndlovu-Gatsheni, 2020).

The planetary impacts of COVID-19

On a broader scale, the coronavirus pandemic hit the world at a time when it was trying to recover from the global financial crisis of 2008–2009, which affected Europe and North America hard. While the world was grappling with COVID-19, Russia invaded Ukraine. Taken together, these developments have negative impacts mainly on economies of both the developed Global North and the developing Global South. This is the case because of the increased interdependencies of the economies of the world facilitated by globalisation. That considered, the outbreak of coronavirus and the way it caught the world unprepared indicated that modern science has not yet triumphed over viruses. The planetary impact of COVID-19 is multiple. In the epistemic domain, our modern knowledge systems were challenged as they were pressured to come up with a scientific solution. New vocabularies such as social distancing and national lockdowns emerged. National lockdowns and reborderisation within a context of the modern world that was characterised by globalisation and increased planetary human entanglements introduced new nationalisms and new forms of securitisation.

Differently stated, the advent of the coronavirus diseases, which started in China in 2019 but quickly spread to many countries in the world, leading to lockdowns and the closing down of borders to tame the virus, has complicated and at the same time amplified the securitisation of borders, migration, and the linkage of rights and citizenship to the geographical territory. But as the coronavirus which neither knows and/or respects borders, or the colour of skin, and the socio-economic class of people, hit the modern world hard, this speaks to the very core of the existence of humanity. Beyond this, the question of the closing down of borders on account of COVID-19 may linger or reinforce narrow nationalism in the post–COVID-19 period, and this has implications on the politics of life – issues that animate this book.

As a result of COVID-19, the state returned as an active actor and protector of human life and accentuated its interventionist tendencies. In many countries, the security sectors (army and police) were deployed to enforce national lockdowns (see Ndlovu-Gatsheni, 2020). The human rights violations and costs of these interventions are yet to be fully known. The ironic part is that the national lockdowns were implemented to deal with a coronavirus that had no respect for borders. The concept of the "new normal" emerged as the modern world grappled with how to do things differently in a context of a COVID-19 pandemic. Institutions of learning and education had to shift swiftly to online/e-learning forms of delivery. The aviation sector was hugely impacted as travel bans ensued. The mask became preferred planetary protective wear while the scientists were busy trying to find vaccines to deal with the COVID-19 pandemic. The challenge facing the medical scientists regarding finding a vaccine can be likened to engineers being asked to fix an airplane while it is airborne. When the vaccines began to emerge, a lot of scepticism engulfed the human population around matters of their safety and efficacy more than in any era in human history. The enforcement of the uptake of vaccines remains a challenge as some members of society remain reluctant to be vaccinated.

Vaccine nationalism and the Global South

The politics of distribution of vaccines was very uneven in terms of access, reflecting the uneven global power structures and systems. This has revealed once more the problems of a hierarchised and asymmetrically structured modern world order mediated by geographies of opulence, on the one hand, and geographies of poverty, on the other hand. This is a modern world that was bequeathed on us by the coloniser's model of the world (Blaut, 1993). The decolonisation struggles have not yet successfully de-structured this modern world, a poised gift of colonialism, imperialism, and capitalism. The key consequence has been what is known as "vaccine nationalism", which refers to the practice in which nation-states, especially in developed countries of North America and Western Europe, quickly developed vaccines and began to administer them to their own populations, and this has left countries, especially those in the Global South, without access to these vaccines (see e.g. Lock, 2021).

For the Global South, waiting for the vaccine has been like waiting for the rains. The other gory aspect were the predictions by such figures as Melinda Gates that Africa would be the hardest hit by COVID-19 and that bodies of dead Africans would be found on the streets. This has not happened. These attitudes, and indeed expectations, of many dead Africans because of the COVID-19 pandemic speaks to the long-standing racial and colonial-generated attitudes informing Western political actors towards developing countries. This deserves commentary.

The very fact that Global South countries generally looked to the Global North for vaccines speaks volumes about uneven power dynamics as well as the uneven intellectual division of labour. In this scenario vaccines are developed in the Global North and tested in the Global South. It was within this context that there were efforts and calls by some sections of the European scientific community to test the efficacy of COVID-19 vaccines on African people. A classic case is that of two French doctors who suggested that the effectiveness of the COVID-19 needed to be tested on Black African patients (see e.g. Rosman, 2020). Although the doctors later apologised, their commentary cannot be dismissed as a simple case of oversight or a mistake but are emblematic of a deep-seated racism and paternalistic attitude towards developing countries and particularly Black Africans. In any case, history teaches us that such a dehumanisation of Black Africans is not new. Examples include, among others, the slave trade, the testing of a meningitis drug on Black African children in the Nigerian state of Kano in 1996 by Pfizer, and the sterilisation of Herero women in Namibia by German doctors around 1900 (Noko, 2020).

It is also within this systemic and structural condition that one must understand and make sense of how the developed countries' support for developing countries to combat the spread of the virus bordered on what can be described as harmful, as illustrated by examples of some developed countries literally hoarding vaccines. Cases in point are developed countries that bought more vaccines than were needed by their populations (New York Times, 2020). For example, Canada bought and hoarded vaccines that were enough to vaccinate its entire population five times, and this happened as most developing countries did not have sufficient access to these vaccines (OXFAM, 2020). It has been argued that this reluctance by Western and North American countries to assist developing countries in responding to the COVID-19 pandemic created a gap for China and Russia to expand their partnerships with developing countries in Africa, Asia, and Latin America. It should be remembered that in August 2020, Russia announced the development of a COVID-19 vaccine, Sputnik V. China also developed and manufactured its own COVID-19 vaccines, which are Sinovac and Sinopharm. The China-Russia collaboration led to these vaccines being generously distributed to developing countries (Westcott, 2021).

But how COVID-19 hit Europe and North America harder than Africa has the potential to wake them up from the arrogance of being a zone of human security compared to other parts of the world. At another level, one wishes that those who survived COVID-19 across the world would develop a survivor consciousness capable of invoking a new economy of care rather than profit in which human health is made a priority. COVID-19 also indicated beyond a doubt how connected human lives are within the context of globalisation to the extent that a pandemic which begin in China must worry the rest of the world rather than being dismissed as a Chinese virus. It is these issues and many more that make *The COVID-19 Pandemic and Politics of Life* a timely book. While the book does not exhaust all the issues and impacts of COVID-19, the contributions raise some of the most interesting aspects drawing from detailed African empirical case studies and beyond.

Structure of the book

This introduction is followed by Chapter 2, which argues that the coronavirus pandemic appears to have caused a fundamental shift in the ways in which the state performs its role in providing public goods to citizens. The neoliberal turn in the global political economy has reduced the function of the state to a minimum level of supporting corporations and maintaining law and order. Although the COVID-19 pandemic spurred different responses from states, they all acted in ways that call for a fundamental question on renegotiating the purpose of the state. The state exists as a social contract to provide public goods for the citizens, for whom it holds the commonwealth in trust. Based on this, the chapter asserts that the failure of the neoliberal state to ensure equal access to basic social goods such as education, health, and insurance to all and sundry led to disproportionate effects of COVID-19 on the population in various countries.

Chapter 3 highlights the extent to which the COVID-19 pandemic and the accompanying lockdowns have led to trauma, death, and destruction accompanied by endemic poverty, racism, structural inequality, aggression, and authoritarianism. The chapter illuminates that in the case of India, the COVID-19 pandemic led and continues to lead to trauma at two levels. This is because it causes illness and disease, and second it has consolidated authoritarianism, racism, and poverty. The chapter asserts that the COVID-19 pandemic has brought to the fore the question of appropriate ethics, politics, and spirituality and in this way brings into conversation the present condition of humanity and the need to rethink alternative planetary futures and not just post–COVID-19 futures. That is, post–COVID-19 futures require a fundamental transformation of the present economic, political, and social conditions; otherwise, there are no post–COVID-19 futures if the present conditions remain the same.

Chapter 4 takes the debate forward and shows that the implementation of the COVID-19 lockdowns, and particularly the closure of borders, demonstrated a narrow nationalism which assaults the values of globalisation and human entanglement in the 21st century. The chapter questions why in this age of multi-lateralism, nation-states in Africa in general and southern Africa specifically responded to the COVID-19 pandemic in narrow and inward-looking approaches such as closing down of borders and segregating against those considered outsiders in total disrespect to the interconnectedness of the world. It is this interconnectedness and entanglement of people, especially in an African context, which should provide a foundation for implementing solutions to confront the COVID-19 pandemic. While on the subject of entanglement, Chapter 5 analyses the geopolitical effect of public health measures like the movement restrictions on cross-border flows and regional security in West Africa. The chapter highlights that the implementation of COVID-19 lockdowns had repercussions on other forms of security such as economic, state, and human security in West Africa. These intersections suggest a complex entanglement of the biopolitics and geopolitics of health and security imperatives in West Africa.

In the implementation of strategies or solutions to respond to the COVID-19 pandemic, there is the difficult task of balancing the protection of human rights, on the one hand, and implementation and policing of the COVID-19 rules and regulations, on the other. This is the context within which Chapter 6 suggests that in the case of South Africa, it was difficult to attain the balance between the responsibility to protect (R2P) the lives and rights of all citizens and the protection of human rights and dignity that are enshrined in South Africa's constitution (Republic of South Africa, 1996). For instance, the South African government deployed the Disaster Management Act, 2002 [Act No. 57 of 2002] (Republic of South Africa, 2002) to contain the spread of COVID-19. It was in the process of doing so that there were human rights violations in the name of preventing the spread of the COVID-19 pandemic. The full-scale impact of this is yet to be documented, but as suggested in

Chapter 6, this demonstrates some of the enduring impacts of the COVID-19 pandemic as the protection of human and other rights of people continues to be elusive.

Another effect of COVID-19 is data colonialism. Chapter 7 argues that COVID-19 has led to increased use of and dependence on virtual platforms/spaces and this has consolidated data colonialism. This is because the COVID-19 pandemic and the use of the virtual space for labour activities has led to the extraction of information from people, and this information is owned and controlled by private data organisations and corporations in developed countries such as those in Western Europe. These companies have links with colonial superpowers who have been engaged in the data collection process. In this regard, the companies with rights over human data have control over the people from whom data has been extracted. More importantly, the use of the virtual space led to a certain degree of exclusion of those who do not have access to these platforms and, of course, the evolving labour market. On this basis, the COVID-19 pandemic, and its demands on how people should function have led to the reproduction of social and economic inequalities, which, through the logic of decoloniality, must be resisted particularly in Africa and South Africa specifically.

The COVID-19 pandemic has also aggravated the health condition of some vulnerable segments of the labour markets. In this regard, Chapter 8 suggests that in the case of South Africa the conditions of mineworkers have worsened because of the COVID-19 pandemic. This is because many mineworkers who are Black have chronic health conditions like silicosis which compromises their immune system such that they are more prone to COVID-19. What is even more problematic is that the working conditions in underground mining tunnels provide conditions for the easy spread of the COVID-19 virus. This is compounded by that the views of Black mineworkers are not considered by the mine owners, whose target is profit even at the expense of the health and lives of black workers. To this extent, the Black mineworkers have come off worst from the COVID-19 pandemic and are treated as the dispensable other. This is the basis for the call for the decolonisation of the political economy so that the Black mineworker is not sacrificed for the maintenance of coloniality and wealth in contemporary South Africa.

In addition to the decolonisation of the political economy is also the need to fight COVID colonialism in which African countries are treated in a paternalistic way by developed countries and also used as guinea pigs for the trial of COVID-19 vaccines. It is in this context that Chapter 9 examines how and to what extent the Democratic Republic of Congo (DRC) diaspora in Europe and North America engaged in health transnationalism to influence the health behaviour of people and public health governance in their country of origin. The Congolese diaspora utilised social media platforms such as YouTube, WhatsApp, and talk shows to disseminate information and experiences about their use of indigenous methods to successfully treat COVID-19. The Congolese diaspora has also campaigned against vaccination trials, which has, in turn, contributed to public resistance to COVID-19 vaccine trials and the uptake of indigenous solutions to the COVID-19 pandemic. Therefore, the COVID-19 pandemic has provided both a site of resistance against European paternalism and an opportunity for African/indigenous solutions to the pandemics to grow in importance.

Beyond the exacerbation of socio-economic inequalities, the COVID-19 pandemic has also created an opportunity for religious and other divisions to mushroom within nation-states. This is the context within which Chapter 10 brings into conversation the issue of Islamophobia in India. An example of this is that Hindus in India used the occasion of a religious gathering of Muslims at Nizamuddin Markaz in New Delhi on 13 March 2020 to propagate Islamophobic sentiments by claiming that the event was a COVID-19 spreading initiative and for which reason Muslims needed to be driven out of India so that the country could become a Hindu *rashtra*, or Hindu-dominated nation. The chapter argues that these divisive tendencies in India, in which the COVID-19 pandemic has provided room to flourish, must be resisted. This could be attained by promoting non-Islamophobic, de-hierarchical, and socio-culturally inclusive practices such as non-synchronous synchronicities and para-modernity to create a diverse and inclusive society and nation-state of India.

References

Blaut, J. M. 1993. *The Colonizer's Model of the World: Geographical and Eurocentric History.* New York: The Guilford Press.

Lock, H. 2021. Vaccine nationalism: Everything you need to know. *Global Citizen.* www.globalcitizen.org/en/content/what-is-vaccine-nationalism/ (accessed 27 December 2021).

Marwala, T. 2021. Global cooperation, and not COVID colonialism, is the only way to end the pandemic. *Daily Maverick.* www.dailymaverick.co.za/opinionista/2021-12-06-global-cooperation-and-not-covid-colonialism-is-the-only-way-to-end-the-pandemic/?fbclid=IwAR0Erv0kX78CiKEj4W1oDn72NhDKIPktK4TTw-pi4bTtC6cbzym1LFq6Glw (accessed 27 December 2021).

Ndlovu-Gatsheni, S. J. 2020. Geopolitics of power and knowledge in the COVID-19 pandemic: Decolonial reflections on a global crisis. *Journal of Developing Societies*, 36(4): 366–389.

New York Times. 2020. *With First Dibs on Vaccines, Rich Countries Have 'Cleared the Shelves'.* www.nytimes.com/2020/12/15/us/coronavirus-vaccine-doses-reserved.html. (accessed 10 August 2022).

Noko, K. 2020. Medical colonialism in Africa is not new. *ALJAZEERA.* www.aljazeera.com/opinions/2020/4/8/medical-colonialism-in-africa-is-not-new (accessed 28 August 2022).

OXFAM. 2020. Campaigners warn that 9 out of 10 people in poor countries are set to miss out on COVID-19 vaccine next year. *OXFAM International.* www.oxfam.org/en/press-releases/campaigners-warn-9-out-10-people-poor-countries-are-set-miss-out-covid-19-vaccine (accessed 10 August 2022).

Reja, M. 2021. Trump's 'Chinese Virus' tweet helped lead to rise in racist anti-Asian Twitter content: Study. *ABC News.* https://abcnews.go.com/Health/trumps-chinese-virus-tweet-helped-lead-rise-racist/story?id=76530148 (accessed 27 December 2021).

Republic of South Africa. 1996. *Constitution of the Republic of South Africa, 1996 (Act No. 108 of 1996).* Pretoria.

Republic of South Africa. 2002. *Disaster Management Act, 2002 (Act No. 57 of 2002).* Pretoria.

Rosman, R. 2020. Racism row as French doctors suggest virus vaccine test in Africa. *AL-JAZEERA*. www.aljazeera.com/news/2020/4/4/racism-row-as-french-doctors-suggest-virus-vaccine-test-in-africa (accessed 28 August 2022).

Viala-Gaudefroy, J. and Lindaman, D. 2020. Donald Trump's 'Chinese virus': The politics of naming. *The Conversation*. https://theconversation.com/donald-trumps-chinese-virus-the-politics-of-naming-136796 (accessed 27 December 2021).

Westcott, B. 2021. China and Russia want to vaccinate the developing world before the West. It's brought them closer than ever. *CNN*. https://edition.cnn.com/2021/05/11/china/china-russia-covid-vaccine-dst-intl-hnk/index.html (accessed 28 August 2022).

2

REENGAGING POWER

State responses to COVID-19 and the provision of public goods in Canada and the United States of America

Samuel Ojo Oloruntoba and Kgoto Jan Mbele

Introduction

The coronavirus pandemic appears to have caused a fundamental shift in the ways in which the state performs its role in providing public goods to citizens. Crises of different natures have always brought out the best and the worst in the philosophy and function of the state and how it uses its power. The neoliberal turn in the global political economy has reduced the function of the state to a very minimum level of supporting corporations and maintaining law and order. Although the COVID-19 pandemic spurred different responses from states, they all acted in ways that call for a fundamental question on renegotiating the purpose of the state. The state exists as a social contract to provide public goods for the citizens, for whom it holds the commonwealth in trust. The failure of the neoliberal state to ensure equal access to basic social goods such as education, health, and insurance to all and sundry led to disproportionate effects of COVID-19 on the populations in various countries. The poor, many of whom lack access to health insurance, have been the most affected in developed countries.

Whereas developing countries might have been affected by the pandemic due to lack of resources, the same cannot be said of developed countries that, despite their vast resources, have suffered severe losses. While the state in North America promotes market values, it generally jettisoned these market values in the context of COVID-19 by providing various stimulus packages to corporations and vulnerable segments of society. This chapter examines the interventions of Canada and the United States of America in the context of COVID-19. The literature on the COVID-19 pandemic has emphasised the effects the pandemic has had on people's health and how various governments' responses have impacted on the socio-economic aspects of peoples' lives. However, little is known about how the interventions of the state could inspire

DOI: 10.4324/9781003415121-2

new debates on the possibility of redesigning the state to move away from the current market orientation. Jones and Hamen (2022) examined the failure of the neoliberal state to adequately respond to the pandemic despite previous warnings and preparations for the outbreak of pandemics. Lack of timely response in the United States led to higher fatalities than in Canada. These scholars linked this failure to the market orientation of the state and its propensity to place accumulation of the capitalist class over the provision of public good. Questions then arise as to why the neoliberal state was able to provide so much stimulus and other forms of interventions during the pandemic, the type they have refused to provide under normal circumstances.

Over the past four decades, the state has moved from its traditional role as a political authority that mediates the competing interests in society and ensuring redistribution to one that provides a guarantee for the market in its bid to accumulate on a large scale. During this period, neoliberalism has taken a centre stage in which the state is appropriated for accumulation by members of the transnational capitalist elites, especially in developed countries (Harvey, 2007; Robinson, 2004). During this period, the power of the lobby groups has increased to the extent of influencing policies that favour the market at the expense of the public (Stiglitz, 2010). In the United States and Europe, ultra-right groups have adopted the Hegelian antipathy to the state. In the process, the question of the political has been subsumed, giving room to a technocratic turn in governance (Woods, 2019).

How did the state in Canada and the United States of America act during the COVID-19 pandemic? Why did the state depart from its ontological market orientation by providing stimulus packages to the poor during the pandemic? This question is important because while the neoliberal state is generally indifferent to the plight of the poor during normal times, they are usually motivated to act during a crisis, though not to the same degree as when the interests of the rich are involved. How can the state change its current market orientation to fulfilling its foundational purpose of delivering public good? This chapter examines these questions in the light of the declining role of the state in advancing equitable distribution of resources over the past five decades. We conclude that the philosophy and purpose of the state must be renegotiated to function more inclusively post–COVID-19.

Emergence of COVID-19 and global health

On 11 March 2020, the director-general of the World Health Organization (WHO), Dr Tedros Adhanom Ghebreyesus, declared COVID-19 (SARS-CoV-2) a pandemic in light of over 118,000 cases of coronavirus infections in over 110 countries across parts of the globe. The WHO director-general also noted that while various countries had demonstrated that this virus could be suppressed and controlled, many other countries were struggling to deal with the high levels of infections due to, among others, lack of capacity, resources, and resolve (WHO, 2020). Recognising that COVID-19 was not just a public health crisis but one that affected other sectors, countries were called upon to put in place measures to curtail its spread, save lives, and minimise the impact of this pandemic. Four key areas were then identified as response clusters: prepare and be ready; detect, protect, and treat; reduce transmission; and innovate and learn (WHO, 2020). Central to these responses were the need for countries to initiate and galvanise their emergency response mechanisms, including creating awareness about the risks and about how people can protect themselves; self-isolation, testing, and tracing every contact; readying of the hospitals; and protecting and training health care workers (HCWs).

Since the outbreak of the pandemic, countries have put measures in place to respond to the pandemic and its impact on the social, economic, and political lives of their citizens. It has been apparent that the global crisis of this nature is unprecedented in the modern world, and the absence of a blueprint on how to respond to it elicited panic across the world and resulted in various states reacting differently in their endeavours to manage this pandemic. While there are arguments that the inadequate responses of the state to the pandemic were borne of its scope and suddenness, scholars differ on this point by arguing that there have been several studies which showed that a pandemic of this magnitude can break out at any time (see Jones & Hamen, 2022).

The implementation of nationwide lockdowns, as one of the extreme measures taken to manage the pandemic, disrupted the day-to-day lives of the general public and caused an unprecedented contraction in not only the national economies but also the global economy. In many countries, this resulted in the closure of many businesses, thus exacerbating the existing levels of unemployment, joblessness, and loss of livelihoods. However, although different countries around the world have taken different approaches to manage COVID-19, some with strict lockdowns and others with targeted measures, much is still to be learned about COVID-19 and how and the extent to which different responses have had, or would have in the foreseeable future, both intended and unintended repercussions across different facets of people's lives across the world.

While governments have attempted, and continue to attempt, to control the COVID-19 pandemic with non-pharmaceutical interventions (NPIs), the effectiveness of different NPIs, such as closing of educational institutions, limiting gatherings to ten people or fewer, closing face-to-face businesses, and staying at home, has been well established (Sharma et al., 2020). Other interventions included quarantine, case and contact isolation, hand hygiene, face masks, public education about personal protection, therapeutics (antivirals and antibodies), and future vaccines (Layne et al., 2020), as well as cough and sneeze etiquette and social distancing (Haushofer & Metcalf, 2020).

The study by Haushofer and Metcalf (2020) has found that while these NPIs have often been used without rigorous empirical evidence on how they could reduce transmission, any given reduction in transmission could not confidently be attributed to a specific policy. However, the comparative study on the determinants of differences in the responses of countries to COVID-19 found that various responses regarding the same threat were dependent on the unique institutional characteristics and cultural orientation of each country and that there was no one-size-fits-all approach (Yan et al., 2020).

The social, economic, and political impacts of COVID-19 responses

COVID-19 has had, and continues to have, severe impacts on health as well as the psychosocial well-being of people across the spectrum of society, and the implementation of measures to curb its spread, such as nationwide lockdowns in many countries, have disrupted the day-to-day lives of the general public and have had debilitating effects on the social, economic, and political dimensions of human lives and affected the rule of law and people's human, economic, and political and democratic rights across the globe. However, while not a single country has been spared, the scope and scale of responses to the pandemic have not been uniform, and there have been conspicuous disparities in the ways and means by which different governments managed the spread of COVID-19 infections and in the sternness of their precautionary social controls (Tisdell, 2020). Without a doubt, these measures can be expected to have had impacts on the social, economic, and political facets of people's lives.

Social impacts of the responses to the COVID-19 pandemic

The COVID-19 pandemic has had far-reaching effects on different aspects of social lives of citizens across the globe, and the concomitant responses to it by various countries elicited unprecedented challenges on the socio-cultural fabric of society. Family lives, and social lives in general, were disrupted as a result of travelling restrictions, restrictions on social gatherings, voluntary and involuntary isolation, and hospitalisations where visitations have been curbed. As Tisdell (2020) has argued, the social choices taken by countries have been complicated by the fact that collective responses to new pandemics, such as COVID-19, are significantly influenced by both the dominant political systems and the disparate objectives of ruling elites. For instance, as observed in democratic countries, the controls seemed to have been subject to a political pendulum of public opinion, wherein when death rates were high, citizens became amenable to governments' measures to reduce them, but once death rates went down, then there were usually strong public demand for the easing of those social restrictions (Tisdell, 2020). This has had an inevitable effect of setting off new waves of infections, as evidenced by the recurrent episodes of increased infections in European countries such as France and Spain (Tisdell, 2020).

Economic impacts of the responses to COVID-19

As the coronavirus pandemic has escalated so have countries' responses to it, and with the pandemic taking its toll on humans, as revealed in the number of people infected by, and deaths from, COVID-19, many countries have responded by locking down economic activity and restricting people's movement, imposing travel bans, and implementing economic stimulus packages to mitigate the unparalleled slowdown in economic activity and job losses (Phan & Narayan, 2020). In this regard, Adeniran (2020) has noted that while public health responses to the COVID-19 pandemic have followed a similar pattern of public awareness creation, testing, tracking, and treatment of those infected and physical restrictions (including lockdowns and shutdowns) to curb its spread, economic responses have varied significantly across the countries in the context of their fiscal space and economic fundamentals prior to the pandemic.

Various studies have been conducted on the economic impact of COVID-19, such as in relation to the stock markets (He et al., 2020), as well as on the effect of government responses to COVID-19 on the stock market (Narayan et al., 2020) and on corporate performance (Fu & Shen, 2020). For example, He et al. (2020) explored the direct effects and spill-overs of COVID-19 on stock markets in the People's Republic of China, Italy, South Korea, France, Spain, Germany, Japan, and the United States of America and found, among other things, that COVID-19 has had negative but short-term impacts on stock markets of affected countries, although there was no evidence that it had negatively affected these countries' stock markets more than it did the global average. On the other hand, the study by Narayan et al. (2020) examined the effect of government responses of G7 countries to the COVID-19 pandemic on stock market returns and found that while the lockdowns, travel bans, and economic stimulus packages all had a positive effect on the G7 stock markets, only the lockdowns had been most effective in cushioning the effects of COVID-19. In relation to its impact on corporate performance, the study by Fu and Shen (2020) found that while COVID-19 has had a major impact on the global economy, it has had a significant negative effect on the performance of energy companies in areas with high levels of the pandemic.

Political impacts of the response to COVID-19

The study by Bosancianu et al. (2020) found that the state capacity was more important for explaining COVID-19 mortality than government accountability to citizens. While the study focused on the state capacity, political institutions, and priorities, as well as social structures, it did not find associations between deaths and the political and social variables, such as the type of regime (Bosancianu et al., 2020). However, the study by Yan et al. (2020) found that although there was no uniform strategy on how different countries responded to the COVID-19 pandemic, the institutional arrangements and cultural orientation were the key determinants of the response.

In a similar vein, Greer et al. (2020) postulated that the regime type, be it democratic, hybrid, or authoritarian and other, might play a crucial role in determining how countries have responded to the COVID-19 pandemic. In this regard, they emphasised the need for exploring government policy and politics in order to understand their different responses to COVID-19 and their effects. For example, they hypothesised that authoritarian regimes were bad at maintaining the internal and external flow of good information, but only some were effective at forceful action (Greer et al., 2020). Importantly, they argued that both the internal and external information flows of both China and Russia inhibited crucial information, although China opted for and implemented effective action (Greer et al., 2020).

Similarly, Kendall-Taylor (2021) and Rouvinski (2021) discussed how Russia and China, as the two foremost authoritarian regimes, sought to influence the discourse on COVID-19 through peddling disinformation at the international space that favoured them and their responses at the expense of their liberal democratic counterparts. To that end, they argued that the information outlets funded by Russia, China, and other authoritarian regimes with international reach were using biased and inaccurate reporting alongside "COVID diplomacy" to undermine the reputation of democracy (Kendall-Taylor, 2021; Rouvinski, 2021). On the other hand, the study by San et al. (2020) confirmed that the COVID-19 pandemic has reinforced authoritarianism and has led authoritarian governments to exploiting the crisis in order to tighten their grip on power.

State responses to COVID-19 and the delivery of public goods in Canada

As of 13 July 2020, Canada had registered 107,861 COVID-19 cases (286 per 100,000 people) and 8,787 COVID-19–related deaths (Detsky & Bogoch, 2020). The most populous provinces, Ontario and Quebec, had the most infections (36,594,250 per 100,000) and deaths (2,722,5628) compared to the other provinces and territories, which had reported comparatively fewer cases (Detsky & Bogoch, 2020). Canada recorded fewer than 400 new cases each day from 20 June to 13 July 2020, but the United States, which has ten times the population of Canada, reported 710,002 new cases per day during the same time period.

Canada took various measures to minimize the spread of disease, which led to a large drop in mobility, a reduction in travel to workplaces, and a reduction in interpersonal contacts, and these included social (physical) distancing, which was the most effective method for controlling the outbreak in Canada (Detsky & Bogoch, 2020). These measures invariably impacted on the various aspects of people's lives, including their social interactions, livelihoods, and their ability to travel to and be present at their work places. They also affected the communities, businesses, and various sectors of the economy. In response, the government of Canada has, since March 2020, put in place temporary measures to mitigate the impacts of the COVID-19 pandemic on Canadians, businesses, and organizations (Government of Canada Report, 2022). Interventions were targeted at different groups and cut across support for people, businesses, sectors, and communities. These are summarised in Tables 2.1 and 2.2 together with the monetary values and the duration of the interventions.

In order to facilitate the emergency provisions of these interventions, targeted legislative amendments were enacted. According to the Department of Justice Canada (2021), federal legislation has been enacted to date to protect the health and well-being of Canadians during the COVID-19 pandemic and to facilitate the interventions. These are listed in Table 2.2.

TABLE 2.1 Interventions to persons and their monetary values in Canada

Target groups	Type of intervention	Nature, monetary value and termination of the intervention
1. Support for individuals and families	Canada Emergency Response Benefit (CERB)	Provision of the taxable benefit of $2,000 every 4 weeks for up to 28 weeks to eligible workers who stopped working or whose work hours were reduced due to COVID-19. **End date:** 27 September 2020
	Canada Child Benefit (CCB) top-up payment	An extra payment of up to $300 per child was delivered through the Canada Child Benefit for 2019–2020. **End date:** 20 May 2020
	Supporting families with children under the age of six	Through the Canada Child Benefit young child supplement, temporary support was provided in 2021 of up to $1,200 to families with children under the age of six through the Canada Child Benefit young child supplement. **End date:** 29 October 2021
	COVID-19 Emergency Loan Program for Canadians Abroad	In March 2020, Global Affairs Canada established a temporary emergency program to provide interest-free loans of up to $5,000 to eligible Canadian citizens and permanent residents stranded abroad due to the COVID-19 pandemic. This emergency assistance was a repayable loan to the government of Canada. Under the programme, the government of Canada issued 4,818 loans benefitting 7,878 people and totalling $20.04 million. **End date:** 12 April 2022
	Canada Recovery Sickness Benefit	The CRSB provided $500 ($450 after taxes) per week for up to a maximum of six weeks for workers who, before 7 May 2022: • Were unable to work for at least 50% of the week because they contracted COVID-19 • Were self-isolated for reasons related to COVID-19 • Had underlying conditions, were undergoing treatments, or had contracted other sicknesses that, in the opinion of a medical practitioner, nurse practitioner, person in authority, government or public health authority, would have made them more susceptible to COVID-19

(Continued)

TABLE 1.2 (Continued)

Target groups	Type of intervention	Nature, monetary value and termination of the intervention
	Canada Worker Lockdown Benefit	The Canada Worker Lockdown Benefit provided $300 a week to eligible workers who were unable to work due to a temporary local lockdown anytime between October 24, 2021, and May 7, 2022. The benefit was only available for periods when a COVID-19 lockdown order was designated for the specific region.
	Canada Recovery Benefit	The CRCB provided $500 ($450 after taxes) for up to 44 weeks per household for workers who, before 7 May 2022, were unable to work for at least 50% of the week because: • They had to care for a child under the age of 12 or a family member because schools, daycares, or care facilities were closed due to COVID-19 • Because the child or family member was sick and/or required to quarantine or was at high risk of serious health implications because of COVID-19
2. Financial support for post-secondary students and recent graduates	**Canada Emergency Student Benefit (CESB)**	Provision of taxable benefit of $1,250 every four weeks to students or $2,000 to students with dependents or with disability who were not eligible for CERB or EI or unable to work due to COVID-19. **End date:** 30 September 2020
	Others	Suspending repayment and interest on student and apprentice loans – **End date:** 30 September 2020 Funding to support a one-semester extension for supporting student researchers and postdoctoral fellows whose research scholarships or fellowships ended between March and August 2020. Removal of restriction that allowed international students to work only a maximum of 20 hours per week. – **End date:** 31 August 2020
3. Financial support for senior citizens	**Providing a one-time tax-free payment for Old Age Security and Guaranteed Income Supplement**	Provision of a one-time tax-free payment of $300 for seniors eligible for the Old Age Security (OAS) pension, with an additional $200 for seniors eligible for the Guaranteed Income Supplement (GIS). **End date:** 10 July 2020

	Providing one-time payment to Old Age Security pensioners	Provision of a one-time payment of $500 to Old Age Security pensioners who were 75 years of age or over as of 30 June 2022. **End date:** 20 August 2021
	Others	Reducing the required minimum withdrawals from Registered Retirement Income Funds by 25% for 2020. **End date:** 31 December 2020 Extending the Guaranteed Income Supplement and Allowance payments if seniors' 2019 income information had not been assessed. **End date:** 1 October 2020
4. Financial support for persons with disabilities	**Special one-time, tax-free, non-reportable payment**	Provision of a one-time, tax-free, non-reportable payment of up to $600 to help Canadians with disabilities. **End date:** 31 December 2020
5. Financial support for indigenous peoples	**Addressing immediate needs in indigenous communities**	Provision of $685 million through the Indigenous Community Support Fund to address immediate needs in First Nations, Inuit, and Métis Nation communities. **End date:** 30 November 2020

Source: Authors' compilation based on reports from the Department of Finance Canada (2021)

TABLE 2.2 Interventions to businesses and their monetary values

Type and source of intervention	Type and monetary value of the intervention
Temporary 10% Wage Subsidy	The Temporary 10% Wage Subsidy was a three-month measure that allowed eligible employers to reduce the amount of payroll deductions required to be remitted to the Canada Revenue Agency. **End date:** 19 June 2020
Canada Emergency Business Account	The Canada Emergency Business Account provided interest-free, partially forgivable loans of up to $60,000 to small businesses and not-for-profits that experienced diminished revenues due to COVID-19. CEBA was also expanded to include an additional interest-free $20,000 loan, 50% of which would be forgivable if repaid by 31 December 2022. **End date:** 30 June 2021
Regional Relief and Recovery Fund	Providing over $1.5 billion through the Regional Relief and Recovery Fund to help more businesses and organizations in sectors such as manufacturing, technology, tourism, and others that are key to the regions and to local economies. **End date:** 30 June 2021
Canada Emergency Commercial Rent Assistance (CECRA)	Providing relief for small businesses experiencing financial hardship due to COVID-19. The CECRA covered 50% of the rent, with the tenant paying up to 25% and the property owner forgiving at least 25%. **End date:** 31 October 2020
Loan Guarantee for Small and Medium-Sized Enterprises	Through the Business Credit Availability Program, Export Development Canada (EDC) worked with financial institutions to guarantee 80% of new operating credit and cash flow term loans of up to $6.25 million to small and medium-sized enterprises (SMEs). **End date:** 31 December 2021
Co-lending Program for Small and Medium-Sized Enterprises	Through the Business Credit Availability Program, Business Development Canada (BDC) worked with financial institutions to co-lend term loans of up to $6.25 million to SMEs for their operational cash flow requirements. **End date:** 31 December 2021
Mid-Market Financing Program	Through the Business Credit Availability Program, Business Development Canada's (BDC) Mid-Market Financing Program provided commercial loans ranging between $12.5 million and $60 million to medium-sized businesses whose credit needs exceeded what was already available through the Business Credit Availability Program and other measures. **End date:** 31 December 2021

Type and source of intervention	*Type and monetary value of the intervention*
Northern Business Relief Fund	Providing $15 million in non-repayable support for businesses in the territories to help address the impacts of COVID-19. **End date:** 31 July 2020
Industrial Research Assistance Program (IRAP) for Early-Stage Businesses	Investing $250 million to assist innovative, early-stage companies that are unable to access other COVID-19 business supports through the Industrial Research Assistance Program (IRAP). **End date:** 29 April 2020
Highly Affected Sectors Credit Availability Program	The Highly Affected Sectors Credit Availability Program provided businesses heavily impacted by COVID-19 access-guaranteed, low-interest loans of $25,000 to $1 million to cover operational cash flow needs. **End date:** 31 March 2020
Women Entrepreneurs	Providing $15 million through the Women Entrepreneurship Strategy to organizations that provided support and advice to women entrepreneurs facing hardship due to the COVID-19 pandemic.
Young Entrepreneurs	Providing $20.1 million in support for Futurpreneur Canada to continue supporting young entrepreneurs across Canada who are facing challenges due to COVID-19.
Supporting Black-Led Business Organizations Through the National Ecosystem Fund	Investing up to $53 million to develop and implement the National Ecosystem Fund to support Black-led business organizations' access to funding and capital, mentorship, financial planning services, and business training. **End date:** 21 December 2020
Relief Measures for Indigenous Businesses	Providing $306.8 million in funding to help small and medium-sized indigenous businesses and to support Aboriginal financial institutions that offer to finance to these businesses. **End date:** 30 June 2021
Supporting the Indigenous Tourism Industry	A stimulus development fund that provided $16 million to support the indigenous tourism industry. **End date**: still ongoing

Source: Authors' compilation based on reports from the Department of Finance Canada (2021)

Money spent on the interventions and laws enacted to back up the interventions in Canada

Canada is part of the global pandemic response and invested more than $2 billion to fight and address the virus, according to Finance Canada (2021). Canada is a founding member of the Access to COVID-19 Tools (ACT) Accelerator and COVID-19 Vaccines Global Access Facility (COVAX) and plays a vital role in advanced market commitment. To overcome COVID-19 globally, Global Affairs Canada was set to receive up to $375 million in 2021–2022 to support Canada's international COVID-19 response, focusing on developing nations' health needs.

The Canadian government paid for all vaccinations and ensured that they were free to all Canadians. Additionally, the government coordinated the distribution with all provinces and territories, providing nationwide logistical support, warehousing services, and vaccine rollout programmes (Department of Finance, 2021). Waiving tariffs on certain medical goods and supporting critical health care system needs and mitigation efforts were put in place in order to strengthen the vaccination drive and to ensure the rollout of the vaccination efforts. Furthermore, the government tabled legislation on 25 March 2021 to offer a one-time payment of up to $1 billion per capita to the provinces and territories to help deliver shots into arms as rapidly as feasible (Department of Finance, 2021). This was in addition to the $9 billion for vaccinations, medicines, and overseas aid. Other legislative amendments were enacted in order to back up the interventions and to ensure that the regulatory framework was not a hindrance to the concerted efforts on the part of the state to intervene and safeguard both the lives and the livelihoods of the people as well as to stimulate the economy.

An analysis of this wide range of interventions reveals the character of the state in Canada at the time of pandemic. Although the country prides itself as a socially inclusive and democratic state, its responses to the pandemic do not reflect its usual character in times of stability. In particular, the targeted interventions to various minority and vulnerable groups are what should have been done before the pandemic struck. Thus, the various interventions noted earlier were not carried out because of a new orientation of the state to be more inclusive but as a means of protecting and preserving the existing order in which the state guarantees the market. While the state can be commended for the ways in which it acted swiftly to order personal protection equipment and provided free vaccines to citizens, it important to restate that the market orientation that led to the relocation of companies from Canada to Asian countries, which led to the importation of the pandemic-related materials, calls for a new form of engagement between the state and the private sector. Additionally, there is a need for a new form of engagement with the minority and vulnerable segments of the population who have been affected by the rampaging forces of the market through being locked into low wages and a lack of access to comprehensive health insurance.

State responses to COVID-19 and the delivery of public goods in the USA

The U.S. Department of the Treasury (2022a) affirmed that the COVID-19 public health crisis and resulting economic crisis created a variety of challenges for families across the country and changed the way people live and work. In response, the U.S. Department of the Treasury (2022a) provided critical assistance to individuals and their families, ensuring people have the opportunity to keep their families safe and thriving at work and at home. These are summarised in

Table 2.3 and include economic impact payments, unemployment compensation, a child tax credit, and emergency rental assistance. COVID-19 and the resulting economic crisis also caused obstacles for small, micro, and solo companies nationwide (U.S. Department of the Treasury, 2022b). The U.S. Department of the Treasury (2022b) was helping small businesses around the country by deploying financing and support to help them recover. The support included tax credit programmes, emergency capital investment, and pay check protection, and these are summarised in Table 2.3.

Similarly, COVID-19's public health problem and associated economic crises have strained state, local, and federal administrations. The U.S. Department of the Treasury (2022c) has been providing relief to state, local, and tribal governments so they can continue to improve public health and establish the framework for a successful and equitable economic recovery. These interventions are summarised in Tables, 2.3, 2.4, and 2.5.

TABLE 2.3 Interventions to persons and their monetary value in the USA

Target groups	Type of intervention	Nature and monetary value of the intervention
Assistance for American Families and Workers	Economic Impact Payments	The Treasury Department, the Bureau of the Fiscal Service, and the Internal Revenue Service (IRS) rapidly sent out three rounds of direct relief payments during the COVID-19 crisis, and payments from the third round continue to be disbursed to Americans. Up to $1,200 per adult for eligible individuals and $500 per qualifying child under age 17.
	Unemployment Compensation	The American Rescue Plan extended employment assistance, starting in March 2021 and waived some federal taxes on unemployment benefits to assist those who lost work due to the COVID-19 crisis. First $10,200 of unemployment benefits received in 2020 by individuals with adjusted gross incomes less than $150,000.
	Child Tax Credit	The American Rescue Plan increased the child tax credit and expanded its coverage to better assist families who care for children. Increased from $2,000 to $3,600 for qualifying children under age 6 and $3,000 for other qualifying children under age 18.
	Emergency Rental Assistance	The Emergency Rental Assistance programme made funding available to government entities to assist households that are unable to pay rent or utilities.

Source: Authors' compilation based on reports from the U.S. Department of the Treasury (2022a)

TABLE 2.4 Interventions to businesses and their monetary value in the USA

Type of intervention	Nature, and monetary value of the intervention
Small Business Tax Credit Programs	The American Rescue Plan extended a number of critical tax benefits, particularly the Employee Retention Credit and Paid Leave Credit, to small businesses.
	EMPLOYEE RETENTION CREDIT
	The American Rescue Plan extends the availability of the Employee Retention Credit for small businesses through December 2021 and allows businesses to offset their current payroll tax liabilities by up to $7,000 per employee per quarter. This credit of up to $28,000 per employee for 2021 is available to small businesses who have seen their revenues decline, or even been temporarily shuttered, due to COVID.
	PAID LEAVE CREDIT
	The American Rescue Plan extends through September 2021 the availability of Paid Leave Credits for small and midsize businesses that offer paid leave to employees who may take leave due to illness, quarantine, or caregiving. Businesses can take dollar-for-dollar tax credits equal to wages of up to $5,000 if they offer paid leave to employees who are sick or quarantining.
Emergency Capital Investment Program	Supporting the efforts of low- and moderate-income community financial institutions.
	Established by the Consolidated Appropriations Act, 2021, the Emergency Capital Investment Program (ECIP) was created to encourage low- and moderate-income community financial institutions to augment their efforts to support small businesses and consumers in their communities.
	Under the program, the Treasury Department will provide up to $9 billion in capital directly to depository institutions that are certified Community Development Financial Institutions (CDFIs) or minority depository institutions (MDIs) to, among other things, provide loans, grants, and forbearance for small businesses, minority-owned businesses, and consumers, especially in low-income and underserved communities, that may be disproportionately impacted by the economic effects of the COVID-19 pandemic. The Treasury Department will set aside $2 billion for CDFIs and MDIs with less than $500 million in assets and an additional $2 billion for CDFIs and MDIs with less than $2 billion in assets.

Paycheck Protection Program	The Paycheck Protection Program is providing small businesses with the resources they need to maintain their payroll, hire back employees who may have been laid off, and cover applicable overhead.

SMALL BUSINESS PAYCHECK PROTECTION PROGRAM

The Paycheck Protection Program established by the CARES Act is implemented by the Small Business Administration with support from the Department of the Treasury. This program provides small businesses with funds to pay up to eight weeks of payroll costs, including benefits. Funds can also be used to pay interest on mortgages, rent, and utilities.

The Paycheck Protection Program prioritises millions of Americans employed by small businesses by authorising up to $659 billion toward job retention and certain other expenses.

Small businesses and eligible non-profit organizations, veterans organizations, and tribal businesses described in the Small Business Act, as well as individuals who are self-employed or are independent contractors, are eligible if they also meet program size standards.

Source: Authors' compilation based on reports from the U.S. Department of the Treasury (2022b)

TABLE 2.5 Assistance for state, local, and federal governments and their monetary value in the USA

Type of intervention	Nature and monetary value of the intervention
Coronavirus State and Local Fiscal Recovery Funds	The American Rescue Plan provides $350 billion in emergency funding for eligible state, local, territorial, and tribal governments to respond to the COVID-19 emergency and bring back jobs.
Capital Projects Fund	The Coronavirus Capital Projects Fund (CCPF) takes critical steps to address many challenges laid bare by the pandemic, especially in rural America and low- and moderate-income communities, helping to ensure that all communities have access to the high-quality, modern infrastructure needed to thrive, including internet access.
Homeowner Assistance Fund	The American Rescue Plan provides nearly $10 billion for states, territories, and tribes to provide relief for the country's most vulnerable homeowners.
Emergency Rental Assistance Program	The American Rescue Plan provides $21.6 billion for states, territories, and local governments to assist households that are unable to pay rent and utilities due to the COVID-19 crisis.
State Small Business Credit Initiative	The American Rescue Plan provides $10 billion to state and tribal governments to fund small business credit expansion initiatives.
Coronavirus Relief Fund	Through the Coronavirus Relief Fund, the CARES Act provides for payments to state, local, and tribal governments navigating the impact of the COVID-19 outbreak. The CARES Act established the $150 billion Coronavirus Relief Fund.
The Local Assistance and Tribal Consistency Fund	The Local Assistance and Tribal Consistency Fund is a general revenue enhancement programme that provides additional assistance to eligible revenue-sharing counties and eligible tribal governments.
	The American Rescue Plan appropriated $2 billion to the Treasury Department across fiscal years 2022 and 2023 to provide payments to eligible revenue-sharing counties and eligible tribal governments for use on any governmental purpose except for a lobbying activity. Specifically, the American Rescue Plan reserves $250 million to allocate and pay to eligible tribal governments for fiscal years 2022 and 2023 and reserves $750 million to allocate and pay to eligible revenue-sharing counties for fiscal years 2022 and 2023. Under this programme, recipients have broad discretion on uses of funds, similar to the ways in which they may use funds generated from their own revenue sources.

Source: Authors' compilation based on reports from the U.S. Department of the Treasury (2022c)

Money spent on the interventions and laws enacted to back up the interventions in the USA

Estimates of direct public spending on the development and manufacturing of COVID-19 vaccines vary considerably based on the range of sources examined and the timing of data collection. Recent estimates from the Congressional Research

Service (2021), the Government Accountability Office (2020), and Brown and Bollyky (2021), along with data on the Global Healthcare Innovation Alliance Accelerator (GHIAA) and Devex websites, provide government spending estimates of between $18 billion and $23 billion. Most recently, the Congressional Budget Office (2021) estimated that the Biomedical Research and Development Authority (BARDA) alone has spent $19.3 billion on COVID-19 vaccine development. In addition, Lisa Cornish projected $39.5 billion in U.S. spending. As outlined earlier, specific legislative amendments were enacted, including those that are enumerated in Table 2.6. These were to ensure that the legal frameworks were created to give effect to these interventions.

The intervention by the United States also reflects the nature and the character of the state. At the epicentre of neoliberalism, the United States has emphasised the market above the public good through reducing regulations, reducing taxes, and increasing technocratic orientation in governance. Under President Donald Trump, the hegemony of market ideas was complemented by a denial of science. The latter made the initial response to COVID-19 to be tardy. The disproportionate manner in which Blacks and other minorities in the United States were represented also reflected the legacy of racial policies aimed at disempowering these demographic groups. While the various social interventions and stimulus packages contributed to easing the pain of the pandemic, they did not go far enough to addressing the foundational fault lines of the neoliberal state. This leads to the next section, where we re-examine how the state can be imagined to redirect its focus and policies towards fulfilling its purpose of balancing competing interests and redistribution within the society. That ideology's common agenda consists in deregulating national economies, liberalising trade practices, creating a single global market, and facilitating the free movement of commodities and capital beyond national boundaries.

Reengaging the power of the state for public goods

There is no consensus on the role of the state in contemporary times. Both the left and right intellectual tradition distrust the state. The right tries to delegitimise the state through its subordination to the logic of the market. The left sees the state as an instrument of oppression in the hands of the bourgeoisie. As part of the superstructure, the state protects the dominant class's interest as the owners of the means of production (Singh & Tiwana, 2019). The responses of the state in Canada and the United States provide an entry point to reengage the state. Through an intentional collaboration of progressive forces in different parts of the world, there is a need to reengage the state to think socially, not only for the preservation of the existing order but in line with its role as an impartial institution for managing society. Granted that the interests of the dominant groups always predominate, a more inclusive society could better serve the interests of the dominant group. Anything to the contrary is a recipe for disaster, as inequality and poverty would ultimately lead to a revolution that will upset any unjust and unequal order (Polanyi, 2001).

Conclusion

As suggested earlier, the governments of Canada and the United States responded comprehensively to the COVID-19 pandemic, and their interventions targeted persons across the populations and different sectors of the society. The pertinent question, however, is whether these interventions, in terms of their range, intensity, and material value as well as their duration, have had the desired impact on the targeted people from different walks of life: the workers, students, people with disabilities, the indigenous communities, and those that have been adversely impacted by COVID-19 and its devastating socio-economic ramifications. What is apparent is that the state has responded through various interventions. We argue that these interventions can provide a basis for reengaging the state to act more proactively, think socially, and foster more a inclusive existence for every member of the society regardless of race, colour, or class. This also presents an opportunity for intense dialogues on whether the state can move away from the current market orientation. We conclude that the philosophy and purpose of the state must be renegotiated to function more inclusively post–COVID-19 and to be able to reclaim its hegemony within the prevailing market-oriented political economy.

References

Adeniran, A. 2020. Comparative study of policy responses to COVID-19 in LICs in Africa. Policy Briefing. *CoMPRA*. https://saiia.org.za/research/comparative-study-of-policy-responses-to-COVID-19-in-lics-in-africa/

Bosancianu, C. M., Yi, D. K., Hanno, H., Macartan, H., Sampada, K. C., Nils, L. and Alex, S. 2020. Political and social correlates of COVID-19 mortality. *SocArXiv ub3zd*. Ideas, Center for Open Science. https://ideas.repec.org/p/osf/socarx/ub3zd.html

Brown, C. and Bollyky, T. 2021. *Here's How to Get Billions of COVID-19 Vaccine Doses to the World*. www.piie.com/blogs/trade-and-investment-policy-watch/heres-how-get-billions-covid-19-vaccine-doses-world

Brown, W. 2019. *In the Ruins of Neoliberalism: The Rise of Antidemocratic Politics in the West*. New York: Colombia University Press.

Congressional Budget Office. 2021. *Research and Development in the Pharmaceutical Industry*. www.cbo.gov/system/files/2021-04/57025-Rx-RnD.pdf

Congressional Research Service. 2021. *Domestic Funding for COVID-19 Vaccines: An Overview*. https://crsreports.congress.gov/product/pdf/IN/IN11556

Department of Finance Canada. 2021. *Finishing the Fight against COVID-19*. www.budget.gc.ca/2021/report-rapport/p1-en.html

Department of Justice Canada. 2021. *Protecting Public Safety and The Well-being of Canadians: Legislative and Other Measures: Coronavirus Disease (COVID-19)*. www.justice.gc.ca/eng/csj-sjc/covid.html

Detsky, A. S. and Bogoch, I. I. 2020. COVID-19 in Canada: Experience and response. *JAMA,* 324(8): 743–744. https://doi.org/10.1001/jama.2020.14033

Fu, M. and Shen, H. 2020. COVID-19 and Corporate Performance in the Energy Industry. *Energy Research Letters*, 1(1). https://doi.org/10.46557/001c.12967

Government Accountability Office. 2020. *COVID-19: Urgent Actions Needed to Better Ensure an Effective Federal Response*. www.gao.gov/products/gao-21-191

Government of Canada Report. 2022. *Completed Measures to Respond to COVID-19*. www.canada.ca/en/department-finance/economic-response-plan/completed-measures-respond-covid-19.html

Greer, S. L., King, E., Da Fonseca, E. M. and Peralta-Santos, A. 2020. The comparative politics of COVID-19: The need to understand government responses. *Global Public Health*, 15(9): 1413–1416. https://doi.org/10.1080/17441692.2020.1783340

Harvey, D. 2007. *A Brief History of Neoliberalism*. New York: Oxford University Press.

Haushofer, J. and Metcalf, C. J. E. 2020. Which interventions work best in a pandemic? *Science*, 368(6495): 1063–1065. https://doi.org/10.1126/science.abb6144

He, Q., Liu, J., Wang, S. and Yu, J. 2020. The impact of COVID-19 on stock markets. *Economic and Political Studies*, 8(3): 275–288. https://doi.org/10.1080/20954816.2020.1757570

Kendall-Taylor, A. 2021. Mendacious mixture: The growing convergence of Russian and Chinese information operations. *Global Insights*, 22–26.

Layne, S. P., Hyman, J. M., Morens, D. M. and Taubenberger, J. K. 2020. New coronavirus outbreak: Framing questions for pandemic prevention. *Science Translational Medicine*. https://doi.org/10.1126/scitranslmed.abb1469

Narayan, P. K., Phan, D. H. B. and Liu, G. 2020. COVID-19 lockdowns, stimulus packages, travel bans, and stock returns. *Finance Research Letters*, 38(1): 1–7. https://doi.org/10.1016/j.frl.2020.101732

Phan, D. H. B. and Narayan, P. K. 2020. Country responses and the reaction of the stock market to COVID-19 – A preliminary exposition. *Emerging Markets Finance and Trade*, 56(10): 2138–2150. https://doi.org/10.1080/1540496X.2020.1784719

Polanyi, K. 2001. *The Great Transformation: The Political and Economic History of or Time*. Boston: Beacon Press

Robinson, W. 2004. *A Theory of Global Capitalism. Production, Class and State in a Transitional World*. Baltimore and London: Johns Hopkins University Press.

Rouvinski, V. 2021. Authoritarian disinformation: A COVID test for Latin America's information space. *Global Insights*, 17–21.

San, S., Bastug, M. F. and Basli, H. 2020. Crisis management in authoritarian regimes: A comparative study of COVID-19 responses in Turkey and Iran. *Global Public Health*. https://doi.org/10.1080/17441692.2020.1867880

Sharma, M., Mindermann, S., Brauner, J. M., Leech, G., Stephenson, A. B., Gavenciak, T., Kulveit, J., Teh, Y. W., Chindelevitch, L. and Gal, Y. 2020. How robust are the estimated effects of nonpharmaceutical interventions against COVID-19? *arXiv:2007.13454v3*. https://arxiv.org/pdf/2007.13454.pdf

Singh, P. and Tiwana, B. 2019. *The State and Accumulation Under Contemporary Capitalism, Monthly Review Essay*. https://mronline.org/2019/02/20/the-state-and-accumulation-under-contemporary-capitalism/# (accessed 10 March 2023).

Stiglitz, J. E. 2010. *Freefall: America, Free Markets, and the Sinking of the World Economy*. New York: W. W. Norton.

Tisdell, C. A. 2020. Economic, social and political issues raised by the COVID-19 pandemic. *Economic Analysis and Policy*, 68: 17–28.

U.S. Department of the Treasury. 2022a. *Assistance for American Families and Workers*. https://home.treasury.gov/policy-issues/coronavirus/assistance-for-American-families-and-workers

U.S. Department of the Treasury. 2022b. *Assistance for Small Businesses*. https://home.treasury.gov/policy-issues/coronavirus/assistance-for-small-businesses

U.S. Department of the Treasury. 2022c. *Assistance for State, Local, and Tribal Governments*. https://home.treasury.gov/policy-issues/coronavirus/assistance-for-state-local-and-tribal-governments

World Health Organization (WHO). 2020. *WHO Director-General's Opening Remarks at the Media Briefing on COVID-19–11*, March. www.who.int/director-general/speeches/detail/who-director-general-s-opening-remarks-at-the-media-briefing-on-COVID-19–11-march-2020

Yan, B., Zhang, X., Wu, L., Zhu, H. and Chen, B. 2020. Why do countries respond differently to COVID-19? A comparative study of Sweden, China, France, and Japan. *American Review of Public Administration*, 50(6–7): 762–769. https://doi.org/10.1177/0275074020942445

3

COVID-19 AND THE CHALLENGES OF TRAUMA, TRANSFORMATIONS, AND DEBORDERISATION

Ethics, politics, and spirituality and alternative planetary futures[1]

Ananta Kumar Giri

Introduction and invitation

COVID-19 is one of the most serious challenges before humanity today, and different societies are facing it differently. To understand this, we need to understand our contemporary human social condition. With the spread of the coronavirus and the rising death and destruction, our contemporary COVID-19 condition challenges us to understand the different dimensions of it. With coronavirus, it is not only a case of a viral pandemic but also one of a civic pandemic (Horton, 2020; Fang & Berry, 2020).[2] This civic pandemic is manifest by the use of authoritarian means to deal with a pandemic, as it happens with handling this disease in some countries. Coronavirus leads to damage of the respiratory system and eventually an inability to breathe. But here historian and philosopher Achille Mbembe (2020) challenges us to realise that humanity was already threatened with suffocation before the coronavirus.[3] This becomes evident with the murder of George Floyd in Minnesota, Minneapolis in the United States at the hands of the police officers whose last words were: "I can't breathe". This murder led to widespread protests and movements such as Black Lives Matter and movements for police reform in the United States. This also reminds us of the challenges of the conjoined fight against virus, racism, and endemic poverty as carried by leaders such as Jane Addams in the United States who fought against poverty, racism, and the Spanish flu. For Mbembe, the coronavirus is also related to our problems of co-living, such as racial co-living, but also living with other species.

DOI: 10.4324/9781003415121-3

Towards a critical genealogy and ontology of our current coronavirus crisis

It is our inability to live with respect and concern for other species and our mind-less and unconcerned destruction of forests and habitat that have led to the un-leashing and transmission of viruses such as coronavirus, which also questions the working of contemporary human civilisation.[4] Thus, the current coronavirus crisis is related to crisis of civilisation (Chakrabarty, 2020). It is also related to crises of climate and capitalism, as critically suggested and argued by activists and scholars such as Greta Thunberg (2019), Bruno Latour (2020), and Slavos Zizek (2020). Understanding our contemporary coronavirus condition challenges us to under-stand what Michel Foucault (1984) calls a critical ontology of the present, which is historical as well as animated by an urge to overcome the fatalism of the present and create alternative presents and futures. Such an approach is also facilitated by Giani Vattimo (2011) in the pathway of ontology of actuality, which also can be re-alised as an ontology of actualisation (Giri, 2023). At the heart of Vattimo's project is the work of weak ontology, which is a realisation of our own limits, rather than asserting our own knowledge, ignorance, arrogance, and power in a strong way. Our contemporary coronavirus condition brings to the fore our inability to know our own uncertainty, as many critical thinkers such as Jurgen Habermas (2020) and Veena Das (2020a, 2020b, 2020c) have challenged us to realise.[5] The challenge before us is to fashion appropriate public policies of containment and healing based upon our ignorance and limited knowledge rather than what economist Jishnu Das (2020) calls an "epidemic of ignorance".[6] Acknowledging our limits and uncer-tainty calls for a new practice of knowing, a more humble as well as courageous way of knowing, a new border crossing between ontology and epistemology which can be called an ontological epistemology of participation (Giri, 2006). Our con-temporary COVID-19 condition calls for an appropriate ontological epistemology of participation.

COVID-19 and the challenges of trauma, solidarity, and responsibility

The coronavirus creates trauma which is both natural and social. But while this threat to humanity should have led to greater collaboration among nations and peoples, it has led to avoidable conflicts and struggles for power. A case in point is the geopolitical struggle between the United States and China during the spread of the coronavirus pandemic. Another traumatic part of our contemporary coronavirus moment is the aggression of China. Instead of doing all it could do to help human-ity deal with these crises, China has started aggression against countries like India as well as threatening countries such as Vietnam and a putting on a show of strength in the South China Sea. Such aggression is accompanied by manifest authoritarian-ism in the decision of some elected political leaders which is adding injury to the wound. Thus, the trauma of the virus is multiple, as we are confronted not only with the virus and the vaccine but also with the challenge of veracity, as sociologist Jenny Reardon (2020) challenges us to realise. Here we need to realise the manifold interlinked challenges of virus, vaccine, veracity, and victory where we strive to realise victory not only over the virus and nature but also with the virus and nature. This also calls for appropriate construction of trauma in which awakened individuals and social movements play an important role, which can build on earlier works on social constructions of risk (see Beck, 2002; Strydom, 1999). Only with such creative articulation and construction, can trauma be transformed into responsibility, as suggested by the important work of cultural sociologist Jeffrey Alexander and his colleagues (Alexander et al., 2004). Both in India and the United States, we see such critical and creative construction at work vis-a-vis raising voices against both racism and the authoritarian governance of the COVID-19 pandemic. In the Indian context, journalists and human rights activists played an important role in bringing to light the immense suffering of the migrants walking back home or boarding the migrant express and some dying on the train. Such construction of trauma calls for a new relationship with reality and constructiveness. As Greta Thurnberg (2019) suggests in the context of the related challenge of climate crises, we need to think outside the box for this, which would help us cultivate what she calls "cathedral thinking". And here Judith Butler (2020) challenges us to realise such critical and creative constructiveness, where we work with the challenge of the pandemic to produce solidarity and we have an ethical obligation to be unreal (see Butler, 2020; Gessen, 2020; Weir, 2020).

In this creative act of constructivism, writing plays an important role as well as gives us strength to go beyond the fatalism of the present. As Fang Fang writes in her much-talked-about *Wuhan Diary* about the Wuhan lockdown in China:

> Since most of the residents in Wuhan do not have their own automobiles, they had to walk from one hospital to another in search of a place that might admit them. It is hard to describe how difficult that must have been for those poor patients. [. . .] We all felt completely helpless in face of these patients crying out, desperate for help. Those were also the most difficult days for me to get through. All I could do was write, so I just kept writing and writing; it became only form of psychological release.
>
> *(Fang & Berry, 2020)*

Writing here is linked to a new vocation of being and becoming, and it is also linked to a new art of responsibility (Das, 2020; Giri, 2020). To respond to challenges of COVID-19 as well as the related challenges of climate change, we need creative and critical visions and practices of responsibility. In our present-day world, we predominantly move in frames of rights and justice, but these are not adequate to deal with our challenges, and we need creative frames, institutions, and practices of responsibility at the levels of self, society, state, and our international order (Strydom, 2000). While COVID-19 threatens the whole human world, what is missing is the corresponding movement of global responsibility (see Giri, 2022).

Challenges of transformations and deborderisation

The current trauma of the pandemic calls for multi-dimensional transformations. For example, it calls for transformation of nationalistic jingoism and greater co-operation among nations, individuals, and cultures. It also calls for transformation of the nation-state. As Arjun Appadurai (2020) argues, the pandemic does not kill globalisation, but calls for a different kind of globalisation and transformation, with transformation of the logic of the nation-state. It also calls for building new transnational institutions and movements. It also calls for building new regional movements and institutions for economic, political, and climate-related collaborations. The current logic of long-distance production and consumption, which is a direct offshoot of our contemporary economic system, is not sustainable. The pandemic challenges us to build new ecologies of production and consumption. Here social activist Ela Bhatt (2015) challenges us to build 100-mile communities where producers and consumers would be able to exchange their production and consumption.[7]

The current COVID-19 pandemic calls for creative transcendence of existing borders and boundaries such as nation-state–erected borders. It also calls for a new art of border crossing where we can overcome our existing epistemic and ontological borders and cultivate new ways of learning and being together. It also calls for new pathways of cross-cultural dialogues so that we can realise new meanings of death, disease, well-being, life, and healing. The pandemic also calls for political transformation, a new kind of politics. It calls for more collaborative leadership rather than single-person or authoritarian leadership (see Willis, 2020). We see that such leadership which listens to many voices has been able to stem the spread of the pandemic. Also, the countries that are led by women leaders such as Taiwan, New Zealand, Germany, and Finland have been able to control the spread of the virus. This has led to a very important discussion about the differential significance of women leaders in providing creative and collaborative leadership in handling critical crises such as the present pandemic. We need empathic leaders who can feel the pain and suffering of self and others and listen to them, who can work as "apostles of the ear", who become apostolic in their visions and practices of listening.[8] We also need leaders who can listen to the voices of their souls, listen to the rhythms of their bio-regions – biological diversity as well as cultural diversity – and the whispers and groans of our Mother Earth (see Howard et al., 2019). We need leaders who become bio-regional as well as soul-planetary or *atomic* planetary.

A related challenge is also practising a new kind of politics, what anthropologist Arturo Escobar (2020) calls pluriversal politics, which gives spaces and voices to many rather than the one-dimensional nation-state–centred system of politics of modernity. We find intimations of a new kind of politics from contemporary critical scholars such as William Connolly (2013), Dona Haraway (2016), Judith Butler (2020), and P.V. Rajagopal (see Reubke, 2020).[9] They challenge us to cultivate a new political imagination and practice which is less violent and based upon collaborative self-organisation and mutual organisation. Such a politics would rethink the current project of rights and justice and link it to responsibility. While working on justice, it would acknowledge the significance of interpretation in realising justice (Dworkin, 2013). Justice here is also not confined among human beings; much more attention is given to the art of living together justly with other beings, especially other species, what Martha Nussbaum (2006) calls "cross-species dignity". The interpretative exercises of justice are here also not anthropocentric or shrouded in the veil of ignorance and arrogance of the nation-state; rather, these involve sympathetic and radical movements across borders where we interpret life and justice not only from the primacy of the human- and state-centred and capital-centred rationality but also from the points of view of all lives. This way justice and responsibility become multi-*topial* where we move across different *topoi* and terrains and strive to create liveable worlds on the Earth by putting ourselves in the feet and trails of other species (Giri, 2018a). It also involves multi-temporal hermeneutics where we move across different times, where we had a different relationship between humans and nature, a more caring relationship, as in our primal times and in some current primal and indigenous societies around the world (see Giri, 2021).

Ethical issues

These issues of political transformations and a new kind of politics are related to issues of ethics. To live with and beyond the pandemic, we need to live ethically, and here we can build upon a multiple understanding of ethics and morality and multiple traditions of it. In this context, along with many contemporary approaches, the project of ordinary ethics as cultivated by Veena Das (2020b, 2015), Michel Lamberk (2010), and others is helpful where we live ethically in our everyday lives acknowledging our vulnerability and, at the same time, realising our capacity to resist degradation and create new possibilities.[10] A related project is a project of emergent ethics where we work on emerging ethical sensibility and norms in our contingent situations and our location in multiple contingencies of self, other, state, market, social movements, and the world (cf. Quarles van Ufford & Giri, 2003). Such an emergent ethics is different from an emergency ethics, which is imprisoned within a logic of a state of exception and based upon fear and terror (see Agamben, 1995). Another project is a project of aesthetic ethics, where ethics creates an art of living – an ethos of artistic living – building upon both ethics and aesthetics (Ankersmit, 1996; Clammer & Giri, 2017). Our current COVID-19 condition calls for creative works and meditations of aesthetic ethics in our lives, which also involves critiques of egotistic and possessive individualism and affirmation of "social and ecological interdependence, which is largely misrecognized as well" (Butler, 2020).

Spiritual calling of COVID-19

Our contemporary condition also brings us to the spiritual dimension of our existence as well the *sadhana* and struggles for transformations. Spirituality is not confined only to our individual well-being but also our collaborative well-being, as suggested in Martin Luther King Jr.'s vision and practice of beloved community (King, 1967).

Spirituality helps us in our strivings and struggles to live with beauty, dignity, and dialogues (Giri, 2018b). It also challenges us to realise the agonies of our life and then engage in strivings and struggles to transform it, thus developing agonal spirituality. Such an agonal spirituality, which resonates with the project of agonal democracy as suggested by Ernesto Laclau and Mouffe Chantal (1985), helps us to realise spirituality as both compassion and confrontation. The rise of authoritarianism and fundamentalism of many kinds calls for confrontation as well as compassion. Here we can build upon spiritual possibilities in our religious traditions. With regard to the COVID-19 pandemic, we can realise that many religious and spiritual traditions urge us to wear masks, such as the Jaina traditions. The Jaina tradition urges us to relate to the virus as an entity and not just as an enemy, challenging us to move beyond the dominant enemy trope of modernistic politics, political theology, and our current war on the virus strategy (see Fang & Berry, 2020). The Jaina tradition has a practice of dying peacefully, and with our voluntary effort and in the context of the current pandemic of death and destruction, we need to learn how to die and also to live with dignity (Chapple, 2020). This is also the spirit of a philosophical approach to our current situation as suggested by the noted philosopher Simon Critchley (2020).

The coronavirus is creating death and suffering, and much of it is avoidable if we have the right public policy as well as the right ways of living at the levels of individuals, families, and community. At the same time, the current pandemic challenges us to live differently and live with death differently[11] and resist what Horton (2020) calls "radical dehumanization".[12] Modernity has been primarily preoccupied with life, that too young and successful life, and it has put death into the background. We need to learn to live with death creatively and meaningfully. We need to have dialogues with death. In this dialogue with death, we can learn from multiple traditions of humanity. In the Indic traditions, there are insightful dialogues with death. In the dialogue between Yama and Nachiketa in Kathopanishad, Nachiketa is not afraid of death and wants to use the opportunity of dialogue to realise the meaning of life and immortality. This theme of immortality again arises in the famous dialogue between Yajnavalkya and Maitryeyi in *The Brihadaranyaka Upanishad*. Yanjnyavalkya tells Maitryee that the world's wealth cannot give her immortality and her life would be as miserable as the lives of other rich people (see Sen, 1999). There is an important dialogue between Yaksha and Yudhisthira in Mahabharata where this dialogue is happening in the context of the death of his four brothers who rushed to drink the water in the lake without listening to the voice of Yaksha to answer his question. This was an act of arrogance which is related to arrogance of many of us in our contemporary moment of the pandemic. Yaksha asks Yudhisthira, who is a living corpse, and Yudhisthira says: "He who does not worship the following five – 'Gods, guests, family, dependents and soul' – is a living corpse though living normally" (Murthy, 2004). There is also a dialogue between Savitri and the King of Death in the Mahabharata as well as in Sri Aurobindo's epic *Savitri* in which Savitri is striving to revive her dead husband Satyavan. This can be read and realised together with the scene of a young boy in a railway station in Bihar where he is trying to awaken his sleeping mother without realising that his mother is dead after an exhaustive journey back home in a COVID-special train during the lockdown in India. During this pandemic, many people – frontline health workers as well as ordinary human beings – are putting their lives in risk to revive others. This is a creative and courageous act which challenges us to create life in places of death and destruction. Through such creativity and courage, which is shown by many people in saving and nurturing lives during our pandemic, we overcome mortality and cultivate immortality.[13] The current pandemic brings us to both crises of life and death as part of our current civilisational crises. It challenges us to cultivate a new civilisation of life and death.

Both science and spirituality challenge us to realise that the virus is not just our enemy. Human life has evolved with the virus (Tanabe, 2020). But the dominant discourse is a war on the virus. A spiritual engagement tells us how we can embrace the challenge of the virus in a new way, do a yoga with coronavirus, which can become viral. We do a new coronavirus yoga, which leads to a yoga of *karuna*-compassion. We just cannot win a victory over the virus and nature, but we win a victory with the virus and nature as our intertwined story, *sadhana*, and struggles for creating liveable worlds of beauty, dignity, and dialogues for all.

Alternative planetary futures

In the context of our current predicament, there is a discourse of the new normal. But the new normal with lockdowns and many other aspects of our contemporary condition such as authoritarianism and violence is also pathological. It is in this context that we need to rethink our present and pathways to futures critically and creatively. We need to work with and transform both our new normality and pathology and realise, as Axel Honneth (2007: 35) argues: "A paradigm of social normality must, therefore, consist in culturally independent conditions that allow a society's members to experience undistorted self-realization". Honneth continues: "The question then comes crucial whether it is a communitarian form of ethical life, a distance-creating public sphere, non-alienated labour or a mimetic interaction with nature that *enables individuals to lead a well-lived life*" (ibid). We need to transform our suffering embedded in these questions and our implicated existence into healing – self, social and global. As Mbembe (2020) here challenges us to realise:

> In the aftermath of this calamity there is a danger that rather than offering sanctuary to all living species, sadly the world will enter a new period of tension and brutality. In terms of geopolitics, the logic of power and might will continue to dominate. For lack of a common infrastructure, a vicious partitioning of the globe will intensify, and the dividing lines will become even more entrenched. Many states will seek to fortify their borders in the hope of protecting themselves from the outside. They will also seek to conceal the constitutive violence that they continue to habitually direct at the most vulnerable. Life behind screens and in gated communities will become the norm.

In the context of our current predicament, there are varieties of conversations about post-COVID futures. But without multi-dimensional transformations – social, economic, political, and spiritual – our post-COVID futures may not be different from our current condition. In this context, we need to cultivate alternative planetary futures both in discourse and practice. But the future is not only a fact – a cultural fact – but also is a matter of values (Appadurai, 2013). We are challenged to create pathways of beauty, dignity, and dialogues and alternative planetary futures which are not reproductions of existing dead and killing systems and ways of thinking. As Arundhati Roy (2020) challenges us to realise in her challenging reflections, "The Pandemic Is a Portal":

> What is this thing that has happened to us? It's a virus, yes. In and of itself it holds no moral brief. But it is definitely more than a virus. Some believe it's God's way of bringing us to our senses. Others that it's a Chinese conspiracy to take over the world.
>
> Whatever it is, coronavirus has made the mighty kneel and brought the world to a halt like nothing else could. Our minds are still racing back and forth, longing for a return to "normality," trying to stitch our future to our past and refusing to acknowledge the rupture. But the rupture exists. And in the midst of this terrible despair, it offers us a chance to rethink the doomsday machine we have built for ourselves. Nothing could be worse than a return to normality. Historically, pandemics have forced humans to break with the past and imagine their world anew. This one is no different. It is a portal, a gateway between one world and the next.
>
> We can choose to walk through it, dragging the carcasses of our prejudice and hatred, our avarice, our data banks and dead ideas, our dead rivers and smoky skies behind us. Or we can walk through lightly, with little luggage, ready to imagine another world. And ready to fight for it

Notes

1 This builds upon my presentation at the webinar on this theme organised by Lady Keane College and Dr Saji Verghese on 9 July and my keynote address to the second webinar on this theme at Lady Keane College on 21 July 2020. I am grateful to Dr Verghese and Dr C. Massey, principal of the college, for their kind invitation. I am grateful to the participants especially Professors David Blake Willis, Marcus Bussey, and Janae Sholtz for their insightful comments and suggestions. I am grateful to Professor Sabelo J. Ndlovu-Gatsheni and Professor Inocent Moyo for their kind invitation for this book project.

2 The noted political theorist Fred Dallmayr (personal communication) makes this distinction between a civic pandemic and viral pandemic. Continuing his thoughts presented in the epigraph of this chapter, Dallmayr tells us how political leaders manipulate the pandemic in countries like the United States: "Medical experts or experts in medical science are often overruled or pushed aside by political power-seekers. In this way, the two epidemics become one big threat to humankind" (personal communication).

3 As Mbembe (2020) writes: "Before this virus, humanity was already threatened with suffocation. If war there must be, it cannot so much be against a specific virus as against

everything that condemns the majority of humankind to a premature cessation of breathing, everything that fundamentally attacks the respiratory tract, everything that, in the long reign of capitalism, has constrained entire segments of the world population, entire races, to a difficult, panting breath and life of oppression. To come through this constriction would mean that we conceive of breathing beyond its purely biological aspect, and instead as that which we hold in-common, that which, by definition, eludes all calculation. By which I mean, the universal right to breath."

4   We can here relate the rise of coronavirus to the destruction of wild habitats and the burning of the Khandava forest in the Indian epic *Mahabharata*. Lord Krishna and his companion, heroic Arjuna, burnt the Khandava forest to propitiate the desire of Agni, the god of fire. All animals, birds, and inhabitants of the forest were killed, including a baby snake from her mother's womb chased and killed by the great Krishna-Arjuna duo. Tatkshaka, the king of snakes, escaped, and he built a magical palace with the help of Maya for the Pandavas, upon seeing which King Duryoadhana became envious. He then defeated the Pandavas in a game of dice and then humiliated Draupadi. Draupadi tried to seek revenge, which was one of the reasons for the Mahabharata war. According to Irawati Karve, it is the burning of the Khandhava forest which is the prime reason for subsequent violence in Mahabharata, including violence against Draupadi, helping us to realise the significance of works by scholars such as Vandana Shiva that violence against women and nature go together (Karve 1991; Shiva 1989). But while Draupadi took revenge against her humiliation, she did not take to task her husband Arjuna and friend Krishna for the degradation of nature, for the burning of Khandava forest. To complete the story of revenge, Takshaka finally bit her grandson King Parikshit. But before this the king wanted to listen to words of wisdom from the sage and writer Vyasadeva, who wrote the *Srimad Bhagavatam*. In a similar way, we can realise the arrival of the coronavirus from our destruction of forests and wild habitats, and we need to compose and listen to a new Bhagavatam, which is a story of human, nature, and the divine, and act wisely by reversing and transforming our ways of destruction. President Jair Bolsonaro, who was infected with coronavirus, has been involved with the burning of the Amazon rainforest. Now the virus has caught him. And it is out to catch all of us unless we stop our thoughts and actions of burning our forests and other beings and weave our own paths and stories of human, nature, and divine, a new Bhagavatam, a new coronavirus and Karuna (compassion) Bhagavatam.

5   In the famous words of Habermas (2020): "Never before has so much been known about what we do not know".

6   Here what Veena Das (2020a) writes deserves our careful consideration: "How could the government not see and only realize belatedly that the policy of lockdown was directly contradicted by the offer of free buses to ply migrants across the border? And not only that the crowds gathered there would pose immediate risks of infection among themselves, but also that as these migrants spread out in villages, it would become impossible to trace contacts? Why did the higher-ups in the police administration neither think that policemen on patrol needed masks and gloves, nor that one stern order to the effect that anyone found using *lathis* (long wooden sticks) to beat up people would be suspended, or a one-day tour of affected areas by senior police officers to rein in the lower-level policemen might have constrained them from using their sticks so freely?"

7   Here what critical economist Irene van Staveren writes is also helpful:

> "I think if we look at the world economy as a whole, we see that most world trade is dominated by multinational companies, by interconmpany trade. That is because huge specialization in low cost production along very long value chains. The corona crisis has shown us the vulnerability of such massive specialization: the global North is too dependent on just a few value chains for ke products, while hte economies in the global South are dependent for their employment on those same value chains. This calls for a systematic change to the world economy towards shorter supply chains (van Staveren, 2020: 19)".

8 Pope Francis uses the phrase "apostle of ears" in his book *On Mercy*. Inspired by this, I have written this poem which can be read in our journey of cultivating a new poetics of apostolic and listening leadership:

Apostle of Ears
Ananta Kumar Giri
Apostasy
Apostle of Fear
Where are Apostles of Ears?
Marching in the Name of Kingdom of God
Ram Rajya – Kingdom of Rama
Banishing Sita and Killing Shambuka
On the Way
Sacrificing Innocents as Lambs
Where are your tears
Where are your Ears?

> [I dedicate this to Pope Francis and other sadhakas and sadhikas of listening in this anxiety-ridden and apathetic world of ours. Bangalore, 4 September 2017. This is forthcoming in the author's book of poems, *Alphabets of Creation: Taking God to Bed*. Giri forthcoming b]

9 Here as Butler (2020) challenges us: "We would need to develop political practices to make decisions about how to live together less violently".

10 Here what Veena Das (2020a) writes with a personal touch is an inspiring example of ordinary ethics:"I am a realist. I know that I belong to one of the "vulnerable" groups, and indeed, in the triage of hospital beds or ventilators, I would rather that a younger person with more life to live gets priority over me. Yet I do what I can to survive".

11 Here what Ramin Jahanbegloo writes in his recent book, *The Courage to Exist: A Philosophy of Life and Death in the Age of Coronavirus*, is helpful:

> Days are very similar in one's life, but one should try to seize each day by thinking it differently. It is not what we do but jhow we do it that matters. We all live the same life but we each live it differently. This is what makes life interesting. Starting the say at dawn is an art that the birds have perfected. They sing to us innocently and without hesitation, not knowing that we humans have lost the art of living. If we human beings keep our faith in life, if we believe in living with equal faith, we will know how to continue to live like the rest of the natural world. It is by a mathematical point only that we are alive today, but mathematicians don't know how to listen to the birds singing. We may not be able to give meaning to our lives with calculus or trigonometry, but we can certainly maintain ourselves on this earth by living according to the dictates of wisdom. To be wise is not merely to follow the path of reason. Many people are capable of common sense, without being necessarily wise. To be wise is to see the cruelty of fate, but also to be able to surpass it. (Jahanbegloo, 2020: 1)
>
> This helps helps us in living differently and to creatively overcome the cruelty of fate during our tryst with the coronavirus, each other, and the world.

12 Following Horton's epigraph about this, here what he writes is also challenging: "At press conference after press conference, government ministers and their medical and scientific advisors described the deaths of their neighbors as 'unfortunate'. But these were not unfortunate deaths. They were not unlucky, inappropriate or even regrettable. Every death was evidence of systematic government misconduct – reckless acts of omission that constituted breaches in the duties of public office".

13 Living with fragility during this coronavirus pandemic also is an invitation for us to cultivate our immortality with and beyond our mortality, which becomes our source of hope.
Here we can draw inspiration from Sri Aurobindos's epic *Savitri*:

> Born of its amour with eternity
> Our spirits break free from their environment.
> The future brings its face of miracle near,
> Its godhead looks at us with present eyes;
> Acts deemed impossible grow natural;
> We feel the hero's immortality;
> The courage and the strength death cannot touch
> Awake in limbs that are mortal, hearts that fail;
> We move by the rapid impulse of a will
> That scorns the tardy trudge of mortal time.
> These promptings come not from an alien Sphere:
> Ourselves are citizens of that mother State.
>
> (Sri Aurobindo, 1993: 262)

References

Agamben, G. 1995. *Homo Sacer: Sovereign Power and Bare Life*. Stanford: Stanford University Press.

Alexander, J., Eyerman, R., Giesen, B. and Smelser, N. J. 2004. *Cultural Trauma and Collective Identity*. Berkeley: University of California Press.

Ankersmit, F.R. 1996. *Aesthetic Politics: Political Philosophy Beyond Fact and Value*. Stanford: Stanford University Press.

Appadurai, A. 2013. *Future as a Cultural Fact*. London: Verso.

Appadurai, A. 2020. Corona virus won't kill globalization but it will look different after the pandemic. *TIME*, May 19.

Beck, U. 2002. *Risk Society: Towards a New Modernity*. London: Sage.

Bhatt, E. 2015. *Anubandh: Building Hundred Mile Communities*. Ahmedabad: Navjivan Trust.

Butler, J. 2020. *The Force of Non-Violence: The Ethical in the Political*. London: Verso.

Chakrabarty, D. 2020. How the pandemic expands our vision of history. *Inaugural Lecture at the International Webinar Series, Writing Post-Pandemic Life World: Society, Cultural Materialities and Practices*. Department of History, Ravenshaw University, July 8.

Chapple, C. 2020. The World's religions in a time of pandemic. *ISJS-TRANSACTIONS: A Quarterly Referred Online Journal on Jainism*, 4(2): 1–6.

Clammer, J. and Giri, A. K. (eds.). 2017. *The Aesthetics of Development: Art, Culture and Social Transformations*. New York: Palgrave Macmillan.

Connolly, W. E. 2013. *The Fragility of Things: Self-Organizing Processes, Neoliberal Fantasies and Democratic Activism*. Durham: Duke University Press.

Critchley, S. 2020. To philosophize is to learn how to die. *New York Times*, April 11.

Das, C. R. 2020. *The Essays of Chitta Ranjan Das on Literature, Culture and Society: ON the Side of Life in Spite of*. New Castle Upon Tyne: Cambridge Scholars Press.

Das, J. 2020. India's response to corona virus can't be based on existing epidemiological models. *The Print*, 6 April.

Das, V. 2015. *Affliction: Health, Disease, Poverty*. New York: Fordham University Press.

Das, V. 2020a. Facing COVID-19: My land of neither hope nor despair. American Ethnologist. In *COVID-19 and Student-Focused Concerns: Threats and Possibilities*, edited by Veena Das and Naveeda Khan (*American Anthropologist* website, May 1).

Das, V. 2020b. What does ordinary ethics look like? In *Four Lectures on Ethics: Anthropological Perspectives*, edited by Michel Lambek et al. Chicago: HAU Books.

Das, V. 2020c. Corona policy must factor in scientific uncertainty. *Deccan Herald*, May 24.

Dworkin, R. 2013. *Justice for Hedgehogs*. Cambridge: Harvard University Press.

Escobar, A. 2020. *Pluriversal Politics: The Real and the Possible*. Durham: Duke University Press.

Fang, F. and Michael, B. 2020. *Wuhan Diary: Dispatches from a Quarantined City*. New York: Harper Collins.

Foucault, M. 1984. What is Enlightenment? In *Foucault Reader*. London: Penguin

Gessen, M. 2020. Judith butler wants us to reshape our rage. *The New Yorker*, February 9.

Giri, A. K. 2006. Creative social research: Rethinking theories and methods and the calling of an ontological epistemology of participation. *Dialectical Anthropology*, 30(3–4): 227–271.

Giri, A. K. 2018a. With and beyond epistemologies of the south: Ontological epistemology of participation, Multi-topial hermeneutics, and the contemporary challenges of planetary realizations. *Chennai, Madras Institute of Development Studies: Working Paper*.

Giri, A. K. (ed.). 2018b. *Practical Spirituality and Human Development: Transformations in Religions and Societies*. New York: Palgrave Macmillan.

Giri, A. K. 2020. Writing Post-Pandemic Life Worlds and Living Words: Ethics, Politics and Spirituality and Alternative Planetary Futures. *Paper presented at the International Webinar, "Writing Post-Pandemic Life World: Society, Cultural Materialities and Practices."* Department of History, Ravenshaw University, Cuttack, 22 July.

Giri, A. K. 2021. Evolutionity and the calling of evolutionary suffering and evolutionary flourishing: Dialogue among epochs and cultivating new pathways of planetary realizations. *International Journal of Philosophy*, 9(3): 154–161.

Giri, A. K. 2022. *Alphabets of Creation: Taking God to Bed*. A Book of Poems. Delhi: Authors Press.

Giri, A. K. 2023. *The Calling of Global Responsibility: New Initiatives in Justice, Dialogues and Planetary Realizations*. London: Routledge.

Habermas, J. 2020. "Never before has so much been known about what we don't know: Interview with markus schwering. *Frankfurter Rundschau*, April 11.

Haraway, D. 2016. *Staying with Trouble: Making Kin in the Chthuluscence*. Durham: Duke University Press.

Honneth, A. 2007. *Disrespect: Normative Foundations of Critical Theory*. Cambridge: Polity Press.

Horton, R. 2020. *The COVID-19 Catastrophe: What's Gone Wrong and How To Stop it Happening Again*. Cambridge: Polity Press.

Howard, S. et al. 2019. Perspectives on bioregional urbanism: transformative harmony with living systems. In *Transformative Harmony*, edited by Ananta Kumar Giri, pp. 317–358. Delhi: Studera Press.

Jahanbegloo, R. 2020. *The Courage to Exist: A Philosophy of Life and Death in the Age of Coronavirus*. Hyderabad: Orient Blackswan.

Karve, I. 1991 [1969]. *Yuganta: The End of an Epoch*. Hyderabad: Disha Books.

King, M. L. Jr. 1967. *Where Do We Go From Here: Chaos or Community?* Boston: Beacon Press.

Laclau, E. and Chantal, M. 1985. *Hegemony and Socialist Strategy*. London: Verso.

Lamberk, M. (ed.) 2010. *Ordinary Ethics: Anthropology, Language, and Action*. New York: Fordham Press.

Latour, B. 2020. Is this a dress rehearsal? *In the Moment, Critical Inquiry*, March 26.

Mbembe, A. 2020. The universal right to breathe. *In the Moment, Critical Inquiry*, April 13.

Murthy, S.V. R. 2004. *The Enchanted Lake: Yaksha Yudhisthira Samvada*. Pune: Rajakiya Sanskrit Sansthan.

Nussbaum, M. 2006. *Frontiers of Justice*. Cambridge: Harvard University Press.

Quarles van Ufford, P. and Giri, A. K. (ed.). 2003. *A Moral Critique of Development: In Search of Global Responsibilities*. London: Verso.

Reardon, J. 2020. V is for veracity. In *Items*. New York: Newsletter of Social Science Research Council.

Reubke, K. J. 2020. *Struggles for Peace and Justice: India, Ekta Parishad and Globalization of Solidarity*. New Delhi: Studera Press.

Roy, A. 2020. The pandemic is a portal. In *Azadi: Freedom, Fascism, Fiction*. New York: Penguin.

Sen, A. 1999. *Development As Freedom*. New York: Alfred A. Knof.

Sri, A. 1993 [1950]. *Savitri*. Pondicherry: Sri Aurobindo Ashram.

Strydom, P. 1999. The civilization of the gene: Biotechnology risk framed in the responsibility discourse. In *Nature, Risk and Responsibility: Discourse of Biotechnology*, pp. 21–36. London: Palgrave Macmillan.

Strydom, P. 2000. *Discourse and Knowledge: The Making of Enlightenment Sociology*. Liverpool: Liverpool University Press.

Tanabe, A. 2020. Politics of relationship in the anthropocene: A search of well-being of human co-becomings. *Paper presented in the International Webinar on Writing Post-Pandemic Life World: Society, Cultural Materialities and Practices*. Department of History, Ravenshaw University, Cuttack, 17 July.

Thunberg, G. 2019. *No One is Too Small to Make a Difference*. New York: Penguin.

van Staveren, I. 2020. The economic consequences of the corona crisis. *Student-Staff Dialogue between Vincenzo D'Egdio & Irene van Staveren. ISS News*, 22(1): 19.

Vattimo, G. 2011. *A Farewell To Truth*. New York: Columbia University Press.

Weir, M. 2020. The pandemic and the production of solidarity. In *Items*. New York: Newsletter of Social Science Research Council.

Willis, D. B. 2020. Gandhi and Aurobindo in the age of Corona: Reflections on transformative leadership, end times and the kali yuga. In *Afterword to Mahatma Gandhi and Sri Aurobindo*, edited by Ananta Kumar Giri. London & New York: Routledge.

Zizek, S. 2020. *COVID-19 Shakes the World*. New York: OR Books.

4

THE COVID-19 MOMENT

Exacerbation of narrow nationalisms and their toxicity to integration aspirations

Zenzo Moyo

Introduction

The COVID-19 moment is going to be a time marker – differentiating *what was* before it struck from an epoch of *what will be* after its containment. The impact of the decisions that humanity would have taken during the pandemic will come into sharp focus once the pandemic has been contained. No doubt one of the major areas of focus will be the retrospective examination of why different nations responded to a global pandemic with narrow, inward-looking strategies, manifested through closing of borders, restricting migration, segregating against those considered non-nationals, and over-relying on clinical science at the expense of other disciplines. What is clear from such strategies was the privileging of not only the idea of a nation and nationalism but also natural sciences without any due regard for the interconnectedness of the world and human entanglements that define humanity's existence in the 21st century.

While globalisation, by its very nature, peripheralizes the usefulness of borders and physical divisions between countries, narrow responses to the pandemic by many countries seemed to eschew this 21st century reality. Take, for example, the lack of synchrony by Southern African countries in closing down borders, adopting lockdown procedures, and what the procedures in themselves should have entailed, considering the interdependence of peoples across these borders. While a preoccupation with inward-looking solutions can be appreciated, there is no doubt that the nature, context, and science of COVID-19 required a deep consideration of the human entanglements that cannot be undone by simply closing down borders and eschewing the materiality they provide. Regrettably, some decisions taken during the pandemic-induced states of emergency, meant to be short-term interventions, may remain in enforcement for many years to come.

DOI: 10.4324/9781003415121-4

This chapter, qualitative in its approach, makes use of critical theory to interrogate these strategies, interpreted as narrow nationalisms, that were taken by many governments as a response to the COVID-19 pandemic. The chapter shines a light on the medium- to long-term impacts of such decisions and uses examples from the Southern African region to show the toxicity of inward-looking decisions on the broader cause of Africa's integration as espoused in the African Union's Agenda 2063. The next section provides the conceptual framework of the chapter and extensively discusses the idea of nationalism. The section is then followed by a short exposé of narrow nationalism globally. In the fourth section, the chapter looks at different forms of nationalism as they relate to the COVID-19 moment. In the fifth section, the chapter zooms in to look at the deepening of narrow nationalism within Southern Africa. This section is followed by one where solutions to the toxicity of nationalism are suggested, being informed by the human entanglements that define international relations in the 21st century. The last section concludes the chapter by summarising key arguments.

Conceptualisation: nation, nationalism, and nationalisms

The idea of a nation is a slippery one. This is because it is an abstract idea that is a confluence of many complex variables – culture, language, religion, law, geography, bureaucracy, and international relations (Tamir, 2019). For one's nation to be identifiable, its culture and history should be apprehended. For a nation to be distinct from others, its language(s), forms of religion, and laws must be distinguished. These processes of identifying, apprehending, and distinguishing a culture and history inevitably lead to nationalism either broadly or in its narrow sense. In his book, *Imagined Communities: Reflections on the Origin and Spread of Nationalism*, Benedict Anderson (1983) interrogates how the idea of nationalism emerged over time. His view is that nationalism originated as a protective mechanism by Western civilisations against the dilution and/or intrusion of and by "imagined communities". Imagined communities here are people who perceived themselves as a social group. These communities grew from traditional religious and dynastic groups to create socially constructed nations. This growth also served to crystallise the idea of a nation, and subsequently, nationalism. Anderson (1983:22) says:

> It would be short-sighted, however, to think of the imagined communities of nations as simply growing out of and replacing religious communities and dynastic realms. Beneath the decline of sacred communities, languages and lineages, a fundamental change was taking place in modes of apprehending the world, which, more than anything else, made it possible to "think" the nation.

From the middle of the 19th century, the concept of "official nationalisms" was developed, originating from Europe. This was a process that entailed the elaboration of a nation, through absorbing naturalised communities into aristocratic and dynastic groups threatened with exclusion from, or marginalisation in, popular imagined communities (Anderson, 1983: 109). Nationalism then developed and was elaborated upon not only as a way to create loyalty and solidarity to a social group but also to broaden its sphere of influence. Thus, the notion of nationalism is an ideology that can be positively deployed to develop sovereignty and unity within and between nations. But equally, it is an idea that can also be used/abused by those in power and their followers to foster toxic relationships between and amongst imagined communities. This is best captured in the following quote:

> Nationalism can be an exhilarating revolutionary force for progress. . .. But we only have to open our newspapers today to areas where nationalism becomes in the wrong hands a primeval force of darkness and reaction . . . I can say cynically, we ought to utilise the potential revolutionary force of nationalism and by our leadership, ensure that the dark side of the beast does not emerge.
>
> *(Ndlovu-Gatsheni & Ndhlovu, 2013:1)*

John Kane (2014: 1), while conceding that it is a slippery concept, understands nationalism as an ideology that attaches substantial importance on allegiance to one's nation as a major political virtue. Thus, within this realm, national preservation and self-determination are prioritised and considered important political imperatives for any nation. This, in many ways, substantiates Anderson's conceptualisation of imagined communities that need to be preserved. Ndlovu-Gatsheni and Ndhlovu (2013: 1), recognising that the history of nationalism has "unfolded and established itself as an ambiguous and ambivalent ideology", also emphasise the concept's protean but strong ideas of identity-making, nation-building, and state-making.

Blaut (1987: 11) begins his study of nationalism with a hypothesis that says, "All nationalism[s] appeal to primitive passions, to 'blood' and to tribalism, and necessarily declares one's own nation to be better than all other nations". This hypothesis, even though somewhat overstated, captures the central notion of nationalism as a double-edged sword. While as an ideology it manages to bring to the fore pride in one's identity and culture, at the same time, it also peripheralizes the importance of other "bloods", bodies and tribes located within similar geographies.

Blaut (1987: 14) identifies two meanings of the concept of nationalism as used in Marxist theory. The first, less relevant to this chapter, designates a set of processes such as national struggle or the national question, in contrast to the second definition, which is given within an explanatory theory so that by using concepts such as nationalism or nationalist, one is actually invoking that theory. The first conceptualisation, which can be used interchangeably with phrases such as national struggle and national question, is used to describe national contexts or problems that may have different origins, significance, or causal explanations. Blaut's (1987: 16) second meaning describes a political ideology, programme, and actions that can be viewed as narrow nationalism, which exhibits a phenomena and belief in one's nationality and identity, such that winning a national struggle or attaining state or national sovereignty "is all that is needed to cure the main social ills of a given society". This belief, in other words, leads one to think that by delinking oneself (and collectively) from other national identities, one's nationhood, or imagined community, becomes superior so as to be able to deal with all societal challenges that may be encountered. To buttress this argument, Blaut (1987: 16) further argues:

> The most often-encountered form of this political phenomenon is the kind of small-nation nationalism which declares, usually in highly colourful language, that independence from the "national oppressor" is all that is needed to solve the society's fundamental social problems. In practice, this position tends to be one of opposition to radical social change within the society itself, that is, within its internal class structure. When a socialist then argues that the fight is against all oppressors, domestic and foreign, he or she is likely to be denounced as a sower of social divisions, as one who undermines the (metaphysical) unity of the nation, and so on.

Nationalism for real-world nationalists, argues Brian Barry (1999: 16), has two central elements that are often emphasised – *blood* and *soil*. Blood is the identification of the nation or people as a descent group, while the soil is a claim to a particular national territory which the descent group is entitled to. This does not mean that the descent group or nation has a claim to a common ancestry, but that it sees itself as some kind of an extended family. There cannot be any doubt, however, that nationality is acquired by birth. Barry gives an interesting example to illustrate this. The common reaction in Britain in 1965 when the then Rhodesian Prime Minister Ian Smith declared a Unilateral Declaration of Independence (UDI) was that of sympathy for fellow countrymen in Rhodesia and not with the oppressed natives. Even though Britons at the time conceded that declaring UDI was a "last-ditch effort to maintain a racialist regime", the whites in Rhodesia were considered by the Britons as "our kith and kin (as the phrase went), and should, for that reason, not be subjected to sanctions by the British government".

Florian Bieber's (2018) conceptualisation of nationalism is not too different from Blaut's second meaning. Bieber says nationalism should be best understood as a malleable and narrow ideology which values membership in a nation greater than other groups, and it also seeks a distinction from other nations, while it also strives to preserve the nation and give preference to political representation by the nation for the nation. For clarity, Bieber goes on to distinguish between latent nationalism, virulent nationalism, and violent nationalism. Latent nationalism is ubiquitous, static, and long term, and it encompasses principles of citizenship, political and social exclusions, and relations between ethnic groups. It can be expressed in a banal manner (Billig, 1995), such as the seemingly harmless flying of national flags, the branding of products, and slogans such as "make America great again".

Through human exertion, latent nationalism can then graduate to a virulent version, which is a stage where the status quo is rejected openly as leaders and citizens seek to reassert the will of an imagined community over political and cultural spaces. For a latent nationalism to develop into a virulent version, argues Bieber (2018), a critical juncture, characterised by a moment of crisis, is required. Capoccia and Kele-men (2007: 347), who critically studied the notion of critical junctures, characterise this concept as an essential building block of historical institutionalism. They argue that "in many cases, critical junctures are moments of relative structural indetermin-ism when wilful actors shape outcomes in a more voluntaristic fashion than normal circumstances permit". This argument shines light on the lasting impact of decisions that are taken during critical moments in history. Such decisions, despite the fact that they are rarely adequately interrogated since they are taken under conditions of fear, often shut off alternative options that other stakeholders may have. Thus, it is often in the midst of these critical junctures that latent and banal nationalism can easily be transformed into a more toxic and virulent version, which can be understood as a response to "endogenous or exogenous shocks to an existing system. These shocks might be ideological, economic, institutional or social" (Bieber, 2018: 521).

At a global level, events such as the fall of the Berlin Wall in 1989 (Tamir, 2019), the Cold War and its ending, and the collapse of the Union of Soviet Socialist Republic can be identified as examples of critical junctures. The outbreak of the COVID-19 pandemic, which, more than any other, deserves to be called a (third) world war, as well as the anticipated scramble for associated vaccines, can easily be the critical juncture to exacerbate some form of virulent nationalism that was al-ready on the rise globally. Indeed, even though it may have been too early to make the call, there were very strong signs that COVID-19 was helping to consolidate virulent nationalism. This raises the question of how we should avoid the pitfalls of the narrow application of nationalism, considering the planetary entanglements that globalisation has foisted on humanity. How could the COVID-19 moment have avoided the temptation that narrow nationalism and exclusionary right-wing politics dangled in front of us, albeit as a (false) panacea to the pandemic? In other words, moving forward, how can humanity, more so in Africa, ensure that only the revolutionary and progressive force of nationalism is tapped into in order to develop an integrated region that is envisaged by *Agenda 2063: The Africa We Want* (AU, 2015)? These important questions will be interrogated in the following paragraphs, however, after a brief exploration of forms of nationalism.

Different forms of nationalism

There are many different forms of nationalism that can be gleaned from the litera-ture. These include religious nationalism, ideological nationalism, academic nation-alism, ethnic nationalism, and civic nationalism. However, the last two are the ones that often get contrasted in the literature (see, for example Tamir, 2019; Stilz, 2009; Bieber, 2020; Bonikowski, 2017). Ethnic nationalism works on a principle that what is often called a nation can only be distinguished by its culture, language, traditions, heritage, and ancestry. In other words, it encompasses the rubric of a nation's ethnic connections, which more often than not, flow from the idea of imagined communities. Tendencies of exclusion within this nationalism are high since ethnic connections are most likely going to be a basis of defining identity and creating solidarity. This kind of nationalism, narrow in its coverage (also known as cultural nationalism), is premised on the belief that the state must privilege certain national cultures that are associated with given geographic territories. In addition to ensuring basic civil and political rights, argues Anna Stilz (2009: 258), the ethnic/cultural nationalists' views are that "it is a legitimate function of the state to protect and promote the national cultures and languages of the nation(s) within its borders". Thus, "[t]he state should tailor its distribution of rights and opportunities in order to protect the identities of its historic nation(s), which can include entrenching their claims to territory; limiting migration to protect a nation's cultural integrity". Ethnic nationalism has been used many times in the past not only to exclude some nationalities in some discourses but also in attempts to nihilate those that are thought not to belong. Within post-colonial Africa, the 1983–1987 Gukurahundi genocide in Zimbabwe (see Ndlovu-Gatsheni, 2012; CCJP, 2007), the 1994 genocide in Rwanda (Jones, 2002), and the Niger Delta ethnic conflicts (Folami, 2017) remain the most significant examples of the toxicity of ethnic nationalism.

On the other hand, civic nationalism (also known as progressive nationalism) is meant to represent a political identity that is built around shared citizenship, respect for human rights, and personal freedoms and advocates for social unity, even in instances where people may be different in terms of race, ethnicity, language, nationality, tradition, and customs. It is a nationalism that has the potential to negate exclusionary tendencies such as tribalism, xenophobia, and anti-migration. As Stilz (2009) opines, civic nationalism simply requires citizens to uphold and respect their political institutions and the principles on which they are based. Civic nationalists, no doubt, propagate liberal principles and attach a lot of trust in institutions as neutral arbiters to any conflict that may arise due to cultural differences. Values of care, diversity, and *ubuntu*[1] are upheld. In a world order deeply entangled through globalisation, where no single nation can confidently claim self-independence and total sovereignty, the practice of civic nationalism offers the best chance for all countries to be able to deal with the toxic side of nationalism.

However, it too, has its critics. For example, Anna Stilz (2009) believes that civic nationalism, as it is currently constituted, does not adequately disentangle the state from promoting a dominant national culture in practice, such as using the language of the majority national group as a medium of instruction at schools. Yael Tamir (2019) criticises civic nationalism for its claim to promote diversity and the associated assumptions that diversity will breed tolerance. Diversity, argues Tamir, opens the door for greater diversity. This is a one-directional development which opens closed societies, but does not consider the instability that diversification brings. For example, nationalities that are forced to diversify may resist due to the social, cultural, and economic anxieties and harm that the erosion of national capital through diversification will bring to one's life chances. This is common and understandable for individuals with a limited competitive edge and are therefore troubled by how they will cope once the goods and services they depended on due to their nation-hood begin to diminish. While these criticisms are crucial and accepted, civic na-tionalism remains the best foot forward in negating the toxic side of nationalism, as will be argued in the sections to follow. The next section briefly looks at the global trends in the development of narrow and toxic nationalism.

Global trends in the development of toxic nationalisms

When COVID-19 started in Wuhan, China, in late 2019, challenges associated with narrow and toxic nationalisms (religious and language superiority, cultural/ethnic sovereignty, majoritarianism, etc.) were already in place. Signs of populist authori-tarian governments could be seen the world over. Donald Trump, having ascended to be the U.S. president in 2016, was intent on going through with his promise to "make America great again" by flushing out some migrants who had settled in the United States. Britain, under the stewardship first of Teressa May and then Boris Johnson, was also pushing ahead with its desire to exit from the European Union, the main driver being the notion aptly captured by Arjun Appadurai in his essay titled "Democracy Fatigue" that:

> It is not difficult to see that the fear of new immigrants (as well as of existing migrant populations) is a major part of the recent growth of arguments against the EU [European Union] in its core countries. . . . It is also evident that this re-sentment is compounded by the sense that membership in the Union represents a net loss for the economic wellbeing in many of its member countries, and that an exit would thus be in their best interests.
>
> *(Appadurai, 2017: 9–10)*

Thus, it should be clarified at this point that the COVID-19 pandemic cannot be held responsible for the emergence and development of the toxic nationalisms that seem to be spreading around all continents of the world, with India, Hungary, Russia, Turkey, Brazil, the United States, and Britain leading processes of political populism, inward-looking politics, and various forms of exclusion – which amount to alienating some imagined communities.

In seeking to understand the source, nature, and extent of these populisms around the world, Appadurai looked at the relationship shared by political leaders and their followers. For one to understand why a progressive "world citizen" would choose to vote for a demagogue like Donald Trump in America or a Viktor Oban in Hun-gary, indeed there is an a priori need to understand what kind of hold such leaders have on their followers. Appadurai (2017: 2) argues that leaders and followers share an accidental connection and overlaps between "ambitions, visions and strategies" of leaders and the "fears, wounds and angers" of their followers. Thus, leaders who are xenophobic, authoritarian, and patriarchal may realise that their followers are "fearful, angry and resentful of what society has done to them" and also share some of their populist tendencies. Leaders then seek to abuse this fear, anger, and resentment during critical junctures[2] within a nation to create propaganda. Because of these overlaps, followers are likely to buy into this propaganda without interrogating its efficacy. Appadurai (2017: 2) further argues:

> The new populist leaders recognize that they aspire to national leadership in an era in which national sovereignty is in crisis. The most striking symptom of this crisis of sovereignty is that no modern nation-state controls what could be called its national economy. . . . In the absence of any national economy that modern states can claim to protect and develop, it is no surprise that there has been a worldwide tendency in effective states and many aspiring populist movements to perform national sovereignty by turning towards cultural majoritarianism, ethno-nationalism and the stifling of internal intellectual and cultural dissent.

Narrow nationalism is on the rise globally as an attempt to fight back against globalisation. But the question that arises is whether or not it is possible to reverse the distance that has been travelled so far in consolidating globalisation. Deep and seemingly irreversible global entanglements and linkages are the order of the world at present, and to assume that any nation can survive independently from others cannot be fathomed. The challenge, however, is that oftentimes, the countries that seem to be sliding into these narrow nationalisms and exclusionary politics are the most influential countries in the world. This is likely to ignite similar moves in other countries if no deliberate effort is done to negate this bad example, and the COVID-19 pandemic, as discussed in the next section, has the potential to exacerbate these narrow nationalisms.

COVID-19, nationalism, and its sub-forms

Beyond the different forms of nationalism discussed earlier, there are also some recent coinages of sub-nationalisms that have been given oxygen by the COVID-19 moment. From these, one can identify corona nationalism (Colijn, 2020; Ozkirimli, 2020; Juergensmeyer, 2020), vaccine or medical nationalism (O'Donnell, 2020; Youde, 2020; De, 2020; Chamberlain, 2020), and information/knowledge nationalism. No doubt the COVID-19 pandemic brought out the best and worst out of people, both as individuals and as nations. In a limited sense, the pandemic engendered a sense of global citizenship that focused on our common destiny as humanity through the sharing of some resources and information (Juergensmeyer, 2020). On the other hand, the pandemic hastened authoritarianism through the institution of a "state of emergencies" in many countries, which enabled authoritarian leaders to impose, under the guise of patriotism, populist policies and restrictions that had not been given scrutiny by those who might hold different views. This encompasses the notion of coronationalism, which explains the tendency by different countries who eschewed the global nature of the pandemic and instead looked for solutions to the pandemic along the national divide and sovereign lines (Colijn, 2020). This argument will be picked up later when the chapter focuses on responses to COVID-19 within the Southern Africa region.

Vaccine nationalism is a phenomenon where wealthier nations can hoard a new vaccine for their own citizens, in the process preventing poor nations from accessing adequate quantities of important medications (O'Donnell, 2020). As Scottish liberal democrat politician Wendy Chamberlain (2020) has argued, people in various parts of the world, whether rich or poor, deserved to be protected from the coronavirus, which Moyo (2020a) characterised as a "global problem requiring a globalised response". The problems associated with vaccine nationalism are not entirely a new phenomenon. It also happened in 2009 at the outbreak of the H1N1 flu pandemic when rich countries such as Australia, the first country to develop the vaccine, blocked exports of the vaccine until its national demands were met. Other rich countries such as the United States, entered into some pre-purchase agreements with pharmaceutical companies and obtained rights to buy huge amounts of doses. It was only after the virus began to recede that these wealthier nations began to donate their surplus doses to poor nations (De, 2020).

With COVID-19, the World Health Organization (WHO) was quick to anticipate this pending challenge and invited countries and non-profit organisations to enter into a pact geared towards ensuring an even distribution of the vaccine as and when needed. This pact, known as COVAX, is a global effort which was meant to pull resources together in order to develop and distribute COVID-19 vaccines equitably around the world. COVAX is part of a broader WHO programme, Access to COVID-19 Tools (ACT) Accelerator, whose aim is to ensure that vaccines, treatment, diagnostic kits, and other health care resources are available to all nations. Through the COVAX facility, the WHO and partners aimed to distribute over two billion doses of the COVID-19 vaccine by the end of 2021 (O'Donnell, 2020). However, as was predicted by sceptics, this target was not met. In fact, a COVAX delivery of 1.1 million vaccines to Rwanda on 15 January 2022 took the total figure of COVAX facility deliveries to one billion, exactly half the targeted amount (UNICEF, 2022).

The dangers posed by vaccine nationalism are huge, and this has been acknowledged by many leaders in the world. In March 2021, Cyril Ramaphosa used the phrase "Vaccine apartheid" to describe this tendency. "Vaccine apartheid must come to an end, because in the end . . . no one is safe until everyone is safe, so all of us must be treated equally across the world and vaccines must be treated as a public good" (Dayimani, 2021). Key in this caution is the fact that the practice of narrow nationalism, in whatever form, may be detrimental even to those who believe they gain from practising it.

Information (knowledge) or disciplinary nationalism has manifested itself in the privileging of some academic disciplines over others in crafting responses to the pandemic. This is aptly captured by Colijn (2020) when he questions the contention made by policymakers that only experts have the "key" to the pandemic. Colijn (2020) observes that the notion that "'experts' and 'science' are leading the search for solutions, and the unproven and biased idea that virologists and epidemiologists monopolize those labels has put the social scientists at bay". In most countries, the lockdown measures that were instituted were informed by clinical science and health data, which in effect tended to eschew the social aspects of the pandemic's impact. This hard science–informed approach not only introduced big and intimidating terminologies but also induced high levels of fear in those who felt ill-equipped to understand the complexities of the pandemic. In many instances, sharing information about the virus became a one-way communication channel from experts, through government, to citizens. In a sense, some of this may have been justified due to the neoteric nature of the pandemic and the urgency with which solutions were sought. However, as argued by Hester du Plessis (in Moyo, 2020c), the hard-science approach in dealing with the COVID-19 crisis was not transdisciplinary, and it inculcated a culture of fear amongst citizens (partly due to the fear of the virus itself, but also due to the big data they were fed and a feeling of inadequacy), and this also led to a culture of silence, since many decisions were being imposed in an authoritarian way by governments. The next section uses responses by countries in Southern Africa as a case study to discuss how some decisions that were taken as a response to the virus would serve to strengthen the toxic side of nationalism.

COVID-19: deepening of narrow nationalism in Southern Africa

Capoccia and Kelemen's (2007) concept of critical junctures discussed earlier is very useful in analysing the potential institutionalisation of harmful nationalisms. The COVID-19 moment, to be viewed as a critical juncture in human history, was experienced unevenly throughout the world. This section looks at how countries in Southern Africa, mainly South Africa, responded to the pandemic in the early stages of its detection. South Africa is of interest because it is not only a regional hegemon but also a preferred destination for many migrants from within and outside Africa.

It was in March 2020 when many countries within the African region, but specifically Southern Africa, suddenly realised the severity of the pandemic. This realisation was epitomised by the sudden state of disasters that were instituted starting in mid-March, with presidents of almost all countries within the Southern Africa Development Community (SADC) declaring states of disaster between 15 March and 2 April 2020. The states of disaster provided leaders of these countries with the power to institute lockdown and restriction procedures, which included the locking down of physical borders that link these countries.

South Africa and Namibia instituted their initial 21-day lockdowns on 26 March, while Zimbabwe's 21-day lockdown began on 30 March. On 1 April 2020, Mozambique declared its state of emergency. Botswana's 28-day-long state of emergency and lockdown began on 2 April 2020, while the Kingdom of Eswatini began its 21-day partial lockdown on 27 March. The Democratic Republic of the Congo only announced lockdowns that were targeted to specific cities, while Zambia did not announce any hard lockdown at that moment (Moyo, 2020a). While South Africa later on introduced mass testing, the rest of the countries in the region could not afford to do so and only relied on voluntary citizen cooperation in order to keep a tab on the overall picture of infections.

It could be argued that if the initial plan was to institute short-term lockdowns per country, then there was no need to synchronise them as a region. But as Moyo (2020a) argues, from the onset, and based on the pattern of the pandemic's spread, it was clear that the region (and indeed the world) was confronted by a "global pandemic requiring a globalised response" due to the time it had taken to spread throughout the world in a few months. However, what is clear from the responses by these countries in Southern Africa, which was more or less similar to other regions of the world, is that the popular lockdown strategy was adopted without any regard for the interconnectedness of the region as a result of globalisation. This disconnection also did not place due regard on attempts to integrate the continent as espoused by the African Union (2015) *Agenda 2063: The Africa We Want*, whose aspiration is to create an integrated continent, politically united based on ideals of pan-Africanism. Since a virus does not respect nationality, any strategy that sought to place emphasis on divisions between nations was not only anti-progressive but also destined for failure.

Thus, the lack of deep synchronisation of strategies within the region (and indeed the world) had the potential to nullify any gains that each country would have realised after implementing initial strategies. Take, for example, what eventually happened when South Africa decided that it was time to open its borders. Its neighbours who share borderlines with South Africa kept theirs closed for longer, with fear that South Africa had high infection figures. As Moyo (2020b) argues, the problem that was soon to confront the region was a forced realisation that as nations, they had responded to a global problem in an idiosyncratic manner that was not only incapable of stemming the tide but also impotent in dealing with the possible re-infections that seemed inevitable. The nationalised approaches and strategies that were adopted at that time were not equal to the magnitude of the pandemic that confronted the region and the world. The emergence of different variants and strains of the virus later on in the pandemic's timeline also made the situation even more complex.

In an equally absurd and idiosyncratic move, South Africa set out to mimic Donald Trump's United States by deciding to erect a border fence between itself and Zimbabwe in an attempt to stop immigrants from coming into the country (BusinessTech, 2020; CNBCAfrica, 2020; Nehanda Radio, 2020). Those who know the history of Zimbabwe and South Africa, as is expected of policymakers in both countries, should have known that such a narrow move of erecting border fences would not have worked, and indeed, it eventually failed, as narrated in *Times Live* (2020). Mukumbang et al. (2020) have also argued that COVID-19 containment measures adopted by Pretoria through the lockdown of the nation have deepened the unequal treatment of asylum seekers and refugees who are in South Africa.

Some government departments in the country, health institutions, and citizens (a minority, it must be said) took the idea of narrow nationalism to another level. They did not only wish to exclude non-nationals from accessing health facilities and other social services, such as food parcels, a special unemployment insurance fund (UIF) extended to those impacted by the virus, and legal documentation, but also actively sought to force them out of the country under the guise that they are taking up their employment opportunities. Economic recovery strategies, poverty, and hunger alleviation schemes seemed to exclude those considered not to belong because they were foreigners. The "put South Africa first" slogan became louder during the COVID-19 moment (Bornman, 2020), which, in a way consolidated the xenophobia sentiments that have been ripening throughout the world (New Frame, 2020; York, 2020) and South Africa in particular (Bornman, 2020; Vanyoro, 2019).

There is no doubt that because of the lockdowns, many people lost their jobs. In South Africa, official unemployment figures rose to a 17-year high of 31%. Loss of employment and other opportunities were blamed on foreigners, and anti-migrant groups seemed to surge in the third quarter of 2020, with several demonstrations demanding the deportation of foreign nationals being staged in almost all major cities in the country. "Every foreign national that came to South Africa since 1994 must be deported", was the demand made at one of the demonstrations on 27 November 2020 by the chairlady of a party called South Africa First (SAF) (Gatticchi & Maseko, 2020). In October 2020, the Gauteng provincial government proposed, through a bill, to ban foreigners from running businesses in townships. The bill sought to reserve certain economic activities for citizens and those with permanent resident status. It would seem the provincial government was succumbing to pressure exerted by anti-migrant organisations, making the decision a populist one (Nkanyeni, 2020).

While it has been conceded that COVID-19 cannot be held responsible for planting and the germination of the seeds of narrow nationalisms such as those discussed earlier, the question that emerges is whether or not the pandemic had the potential to help consolidate the spread of these toxic nationalisms, especially in Southern Africa, and South Africa in particular. The discussion so far forces us to answer this question in the affirmative. This then necessitates the answering of another important question posed by Colijn (2020): How do we achieve the collective good which is self-evident in eliminating existential threats like COVID-19, which does not hold up within national borders? The next section answers this question by proposing alternative approaches that should have been, or should be, adopted to negate narrow nationalism.

Human entanglements and solutions to narrow nationalism as a result of COVID-19

Nationalism has generally been seen as both positive and negative and fittingly likened to electricity – which has the potential to heat and light the world and at the same time is capable of electrocuting someone who mishandles it (Ndlovu-Gatsheni &

Ndhlovu, 2013). In this chapter, nationalism has been used mainly to shine light on its toxicity whenever and wherever it is being exerted. However, there is a version of nationalism, civic in its orientation, which, despite its liberal tentacles, can be used gainfully for the benefit of the less powerful and excluded. This is the nationalism that this chapter recommends as ideal for practice during critical junctures such as was the case during the COVID-19 pandemic. To recap slightly, the practice of civic nationalism does not emphasise the principles of "blood and soil" as does ethnic nationalism, but that of shared citizenship and the respect for human rights, unity, and personal freedoms. However, some theorists such as Yamir (2019) and Stilz (2009) are sceptical about the efficacy of civic nationalism, and the basis of their scepticism is that civic nationalism, as currently constituted, offers a model that is too legalistic and abstract, and therefore covers a limited scope of a citizen's life. While this criticism may be valid, ideas of constitutionalism, universal rights, law enforcement, and equal membership have always been central to successful democracies, and this chapter argues that it is within the abilities of leaders to ensure that these universal ideas prevail.

Governments do possess the key to stop or negate toxic nationalism. Political leaders only need to resist a temptation to abuse people's fears, wounds, and angers as strategies to quench their political ambition to be popular (Appadurai, 2017). If citizens of any country are afforded a decent quality of life by their government, where socio-economic goods and services, such as jobs, housing, access to health, and education are provided, the need to denigrate or exclude other nationalities will not arise. If it arises, the government should, without fear of contradiction, have a right to invoke legal provisions to protect those who are being excluded. Values of universal care should be touted by any government as the basis upon which national laws and policies should be crafted, even in times of crises.

At the time of drafting this chapter in 2020, which was also the year when COVID-19 spread in Africa, South African President Cyril Ramaphosa was the chairperson of the African Union (AU).[3] The policy to erect a border fence between Zimbabwe and South Africa as a coronavirus containment measure was also implemented under his presidency. The paradox that need not be missed is how actions, such as the unilateral strengthening of border divisions through fences, contradicts the aspirations of the same AU that Ramaphosa was chairing. These aspirations are expressed in the AU's Agenda 2063 document (AU, 2015:4) as follows:

We aspire that by 2063, Africa shall:

- Be a United Africa
- Have a world class, integrative infrastructure that criss-crosses the continent
- Have dynamic and mutually beneficial links with her diaspora; and
- Be a continent of seamless borders [emphasis added], and management of cross-border resources through dialogue

The AU's Agenda 2063 document goes on to tell us that Africa shall be an integrated, united, peaceful, sovereign, independent, confident, and self-reliant continent.

Measures that individual countries in Southern Africa instituted to mitigate the COVID-19 pandemic, including the erection of border fences, the non-synchronisation of lockdown procedures, and border closures, work against the aspirations contained in Agenda 2063. Some of these measures taken during the states of emergency, such as the securitisation of borders and the erection of the R37 million border fence (BussinessTech, 2020), seem to portend some permanency and no doubt will remain in place beyond the containment of the pandemic. This, for all intents and purposes, will undo all that has been and is still to be done to realise the African aspirations of developing an integrated, united, and peaceful Africa. In fact, the COVID-19 moment should have been used as a heuristic tool to march faster towards integrating the region and the continent, rather than further entrenching divisions.

Another strategy that should have been afforded pride of place while making decisions during the COVID-19 moment is what has been understood as transdisciplinary approaches. Transdisciplinarity is an approach to problem solving, which dissolves academic disciplinary boundaries when dealing with any societal challenges, because it allows and respects the entrance of all forms of knowledge into the "knowledge production matrix" (Moyo, 2020c). MISTRA (2019) provides a definition of transdisciplinarity as follows:

> Transdisciplinarity is an attempt at formulating an integrative process of knowledge production and dissemination. Transdisciplinarity is, in part, a reaction against the twentieth century occurrence of narrow discipline focus and hyperspecialisation. It attempts to directly respond to the multi-layered challenges of diffuse disciplines, interlinked socio-economic problems, impacts of globalisation, de-territorialised nation-states, technological advancements, environmental concerns, food security and so on.

Transdisciplinarity is a transgressive approach because it promotes mutual learning between sciences and practice, and therefore provides space for the resolution of challenges that may arise between science in its broadest sense, culture and democracy. During the COVID-19 moment, and because of the shape-shifting character of the virus (Moyo, 2020c), the privileging of knowledge from clinical and medical sciences only – was inadequate, and that is why an environment of fear within communities was engendered, particularly in South Africa where several court cases were instituted against the government for some of the policies it had adopted (see Merten, 2020).

Narrow and inward-looking internal strategies were never likely to offer a lasting solution to the COVID-19 pandemic. Indeed, it should have been predictable even early on that at some point, there would be a choice between saving lives and saving livelihoods. How does a government save livelihoods if it prioritises clinical science and peripheralizes other academic disciplines and data-gathering methodologies, or if it degenerates into ethnic and cultural nationalism, where other nationalities no longer matter? Moving forward, the best way to deal with a pandemic of this nature and magnitude is to adopt an incremental approach, beginning at the regional level all the way up to global cooperation. Thus, as Moyo (2020a) argues, without adopting synchronised strategies, the fight against the coronavirus will be replete with false starts. And this probably explains the severity of the second and third waves experienced by many countries due to the more virulent variants of the pandemic. Moving into the future, vaccines for COVID-19 and future pandemics should be treated as a public good in every continent, region, and country, so that all and sundry can have unhindered access to help. Like it has been argued (Chutel & Santora, 2021), total vaccination in some parts of the world will come to naught if other parts of the world remain exposed, and thus remain susceptible to the mutation of the virus that may then be resistant to the vaccines that have been developed.

Social science and humanities needed to play a more critical role not only in analysing the societal impact of the virus but also in informing governments' responses to the pandemic. Thus, transdisciplinary thinking the world over, but Africa in particular, would have enabled a strategic reflection on some issues that ended up shaping narrow nationalism. With the deep entanglements that globalisation has foisted on us, humanity cannot afford to segregate each other. A values-based culture of care needs to be cultivated in all human interactions.

Conclusion

The idea of nationalism has been used for many years as a force for good. Take, for example, the unity and solidarity that it brought during anti-colonial struggles in formerly colonised countries. However, of late, this ideology has been weaponised by some leaders and their followers as an instrument to exclude those who are seen as not part of a particular imagined community. This exclusion, in many instances, is more pronounced in times of crises and during critical junctures such as the COVID-19 moment. We have seen in many instances where this ideology mutates to take the "shape and colour" of the crisis feeding it at any particular moment. If the problem is about economic decline, nations are rallied against non-nationals, who are portrayed as responsible for the collapsing economy. If the problem is about the outbreak of a pandemic, nationals of other countries get blamed more, and even labelled as super-spreaders of a pandemic that knows no colour, gender, or nationality.

This chapter has discussed different versions of nationalism and dwelt particularly on the narrow, inward-looking approaches that have come to give prominence to tendencies of exclusion and the idea that there are some people whose voices and feelings are not worthy of circulation in societies where they live. This exclusion has been visible in the way in which many countries have responded to the existential threat brought by the COVID-19 pandemic, including the temptation to close borders, erect borderline fences, and limit access to the health infrastructure and medication only to nationals. The chapter has further argued that due to the global entanglements that globalisation has foisted on humanity, narrow nationalism, as elucidated earlier, has no place in the future of humanity. While the expression of narrow nationalism seems to be a symptom of deeper challenges that governments must confront, it remains not an answer to such challenges. It is within the power of leaders in any particular country and region to ensure that the resolution of any challenges faced is achieved without resorting to exclusionary tactics.

The chapter ended by suggesting some approaches that could be adopted to prevent toxic nationalism from rearing its ugly head in crisis times such as the COVID-19 moment. However, since the COVID-19 is a novel virus, it is more likely that a lot is still to be known, and a lot will still change. The suggestions offered earlier, such as the prioritisation of the civic version of nationalism, may be used as a start to ensure the inculcation of the value of care within humanity. The ideal of living together harmoniously as human beings should be everyone's aim, and it can only be through doing so that humanity can conquer the challenges it faces, including pandemics, such as COVID-19.

Notes

1 *Ubuntu* is a Nguni concept that captures the spirit of common humanity amongst people. It is coined from a longer phrase, *umuntu ngumuntu ngabantu*, which loosely means "I am, because you are".
2 Critical junctures are key in this analysis because that is when propaganda is heightened and often not challenged because space to do so is shrunk. Uncritical consensus then becomes the order of conducting business.
3 This chairmanship was passed on to the Democratic Republic of Congo leader, President Felix-Antoine Tshisekedi, in February 2021.

References

African Union (AU). 2015. *Agenda 2063: The Africa We want (Popular version).* https://au.int/sites/default/files/documents/36204-doc-agenda2063_popular_version_en.pdf (accessed 9 December 2020).
Anderson, B. 1983. *Imagined Communities: Reflections on the Origin and Spread of Nationalism.* London: Verso.
Appadurai, A. 2017. Democracy fatigue. In *The Great Regression*, edited by Heinrich Geiselberger, pp. 1–12. Cambridge: Polity Press.
Barry, B. 1999. Statism and Nationalism: A cosmopolitan critique. *Nomos*, 41: 12–66.
Bieber, F. 2018. Is nationalism on the rise? *Assessing Global Trends. Ethnopolitics*, 17(5): 519–540.
Bieber, F. 2020. *Debating Nationalism: The Global Spread of Nations.* London: Bloomsbury.
Billig, M. 1995. *Banal Nationalism.* London: SAGE.
Blaut, J. M. 1987. *The National Question.* London: Zed Books.
Bonikowski, B. 2017. Ethno-nationalist populism and the mobilization of collective resentment. *The British Journal of Sociology*, 68: 181–213.
Bornman, J. 2020. South Africa: Rising xenophobia needs to be challenged. *New Frame*, 26 August. www.newframe.com/rising-xenophobia-needs-to-be-challenged/ (accessed 16 December 2020).
BussinessTech. 2020. *A Look at South Africa's R37 Million Border Fence with Zimbabwe – Built to Stop the Spread of the Coronavirus*, 1 May. https://businesstech.co.za/news/government/396733/a-look-at-south-africas-r37-million-border-fence-with-zimbabwe-built-to-stop-the-spread-of-the-coronavirus/ (accessed 16 December 2020).

Capoccia, G. and Kelemen, R. D. 2007. The study of critical junctures: Theory, narrative and counterfactuals in historical institutionalism. *World Politics*, 59: 341–369.

CCJP. 2007. *Gukurahundi in Zimbabwe: A Report on the Disturbances in the Matabeleland and the Midlands*. London: Hurst and Company.

Chamberlain, W. 2020. 'Vaccine nationalism' has begun – but we are not safe until we are all safe. *Independent*, 23 November. www.independent.co.uk/voices/vaccine-nationalism-coronavirus-covid19-b1759346.html (accessed 16 December 2020).

Chutel, L. and Santora, M. 2021. As virus variants spread, 'No one is safe until everyone is safe'. *The New York Times*, 31 January 2021. www.nytimes.com/2021/01/31/world/africa/coronavirus-south-africa-variant.html (accessed 2 April 2021).

CNBCAfrica. 2020. *S. Africa to Erect 40km Fence on Zimbabwe Border as Coronavirus Measure*, 19 March. www.cnbcafrica.com/news/2020/03/19/s-africa-to-erect-40km-fence-on-zimbabwe-border-as-coronavirus-measure/ (accessed 16 December 2020).

Colijn, C. 2020. Coronationalism. *Clingendiel Spectator*, 18 March. https://spectator.clingendael.org/nl/publicatie/coronationalisme (accessed 16 December 2020).

Dayimani, M. 2021. COVID-19: Ramaphosa admits govt behind vaccine targets, hints at stronger lockdown ahead of Easter. *News24*, 29 March. www.news24.com/news24/SouthAfrica/News/covid-19-ramaphosa-admits-govt-behind-vaccine-targets-hints-at-stronger-lockdown-ahead-of-easter-20210329 (accessed 2 April 2021).

De, A. 2020. Explained: Vaccine nationalism, and how it impacts the COVID-19 fight. *The Indian Express*, 23 August. https://indianexpress.com/article/explained/what-is-vaccine-nationalism-how-does-it-impact-the-fight-against-covid-19-6561236/ (accessed 16 December 2020).

Folami, J. M. 2017. Ethnic-conflict and its manifestations in the politics of recognition in multi-ethnic Niger delta region. *Cogent Social Sciences*, 3(1): 1–17.

Gatticchi, G. and Maseko, L. 2020. Xenophobia surges as COVID-19 slams South African economy. *Bloomberg*, 20 December. www.bloombergquint.com/onweb/xenophobia-surges-as-covid-19-slams-south-african-economy (accessed 20 December 2020).

Jones, A. 2002. Gender and genocide in Rwanda. *Journal of Genocide Research*, 4(1): 65–94.

Juergensmeyer, M. 2020. COVID Nationalism. *E-International Relations*, 6 September. www.e-ir.info/2020/09/06/covid-nationalism/ (accessed 10 December 2020).

Kane, J. 2014. Nationalism. *Wiley Online Library*, 15 September. https://onlinelibrary.wiley.com/doi/10.1002/9781118474396.wbept0697 (accessed 10 December 2020).

Merten, M. 2020. Another lockdown challenge heads to ConCourt. *Daily Maverick*, 2 July. www.dailymaverick.co.za/article/2020-07-02-another-lockdown-challenge-heads-to-concourt/ (accessed 10 September 2020).

MISTRA. 2019. *The Concept and Application of Transdisciplinarity in Intellectual Discourse and Research* (Du Plessis, H; Sehume, J and Martin, L (eds.)). Johannesburg: Mapungubwe Institute for Strategic Reflection.

Moyo, Z. 2020a. COVID-19: A global problem requiring a globalised response. *The Standard*, 5 April. www.thestandard.co.zw/2020/04/05/covid-19-global-problem-requiring-globalised-response/ (accessed 16 December 2020).

Moyo, Z. 2020b. COVID-19: A global problem requiring a globalised response. *Mapungubwe Institute for Strategic Reflection*. https://mistra.org.za/mistra-media/covid-19-a-global-problem-requiring-a-globalised-response/ (accessed 10 December 2020).

Moyo, Z. 2020c. The need for a transdisciplinary approach to South Africa's COVID-19 crisis. *Mapungubwe Institute for Strategic Reflection, Synthesis Report*, 8 October. https://mistra.org.za/mistra-media/the-need-for-a-transdisciplinary-approach-to-south-africas-covid-19-crisis/ (accessed 16 December 2020).

Mukumbang, F. C., Ambe, A. N. and Adebiyi, B. O. 2020. Unspoken inequality: How COVID-19 has exacerbated existing vulnerabilities of asylum-seekers, refugees, and un-documented migrants in South Africa. *International Journal for Equity in Health*, 19(141): 1–7.

Ndlovu-Gatsheni, S. J. 2012. Rethinking Chimurenga and Gukurahundi in Zimbabwe: A critique of partisan national history. *African Studies Review*, 55: 1–26.

Ndlovu-Gatsheni, S. J. and Ndhlovu, F. 2013. *Nationalism and National Projects in Southern Africa: New Critical Reflections*. Pretoria; Africa Institute of South Africa.

Nehanda Radio. 2020. *South Africa Erects 40km fence on Zimbabwe Border as Coronavirus Measure*, 20 March. https://nehandaradio.com/2020/03/20/south-africa-erects-40km-fence-on-zimbabwe-border-as-coronavirus-measure/ (accessed, 16 December 2020).

New Frame. 2020. *Xenophobia on the Rise as COVID-19 Roils the Planet*, 15 May. www.newframe.com/xenophobia-on-the-rise-as-covid-19-roils-the-planet/ (accessed 17 December 2020).

Nkanjeni, U. 2020. Township economy bill would fuel xenophobia, DA's Makashule Gana says. *Business Day*, 20 October. www.businesslive.co.za/bd/national/2020-10-20-township-economy-bill-would-fuel-xenophobia-das-makashule-gana-says/ (accessed 20 December 2020).

O'Donnell, C. 2020. Inside WHO's Plan to 'Prevent COVID-19 Vaccine Nationalism'. *Times Live*, 19 August. www.timeslive.co.za/sunday-times/lifestyle/2020-08-19-inside-whos-plan-to-prevent-covid-19-vaccine-nationalism/ (accessed 16 December 2020).

Ozkirimli, U. 2020. Coronationalism? *OpenDemocracy*, 14 April. www.opendemocracy.net/en/can-europe-make-it/coronationalism/ (accessed 16 December 2020).

Stilz, A. 2009. Civic Nationalism and language policy. *Philosophy and Public Affairs*, 37(3): 257–292.

Tamir, Y. 2019. Not so civic: Is there a difference between ethnic and civic nationalism? *Annual Review of Political Science*, 22: 419–434.

Times Live. 2020. Army heads to SA-Zimbabwe border after new R37m fence damaged. *Times Live*, 13 April. www.timeslive.co.za/news/south-africa/2020-04-13-army-heads-to-sa-zimbabwe-border-after-new-r37m-fence-damaged/ (accessed 16 December 2020).

UNICEF. 2022. *COVAX: 1 Billion Vaccines Delivered: Milestone COVID-19 Vaccine Shipment Arrives in Kigali, Rwanda*. https://www.unicef.org/supply/stories/covax-1-billion-vaccines-delivered (accessed 25 May 2023).

Vanyoro, K. 2019. Telling the complex story of 'medical xenophobia' in South Africa. *Mail and Guardian*, 12 December. https://mg.co.za/article/2019-12-12-00-telling-the-complex-story-of-medical-xenophobia-in-south-africa/ (accessed 16 December 2020).

York, G. 2020. Coronavirus triggers xenophobia in some African countries. *The Globe and Mail*, 19 March. www.theglobeandmail.com/world/article-coronavirus-triggers-xenophobia-in-some-african-countries/ (accessed 16 December 2020).

Youde, J. 2020. How 'medical nationalism' is undermining the fight against the coronavirus pandemic. *World Politics Review*, 23 March. www.worldpoliticsreview.com/articles/28623/how-medical-nationalism-is-undermining-the-fight-against-the-coronavirus-pandemic (accessed 16 December 2020).

5

COVID-19 PANDEMIC, GEOPOLITICS OF HEALTH, AND SECURITY ENTANGLEMENT IN WEST AFRICA

Olukayode A. Faleye

Introduction

The outbreak of severe acute respiratory syndrome – coronavirus 2, the virus responsible for the COVID-19 pandemic, is a watershed moment in the history of global health. Studies have shown the correlation between early deployments of public health measures of movement restrictions and the abatement of the spread of the COVID-19 pandemic around the world (Memon et al., 2021). In reconstructing the contemporary social history of the pandemic, scholars have adopted the top-down approach in analysing the biopolitics of health in tandem with the notions of class struggle and deepening of the "uneven" structures of global capitalism in the COVID-19 era (Harvey, 2020; Van Dorn et al., 2020; Pulignano &Mara, 2020; Grundy-Wan &Lin, 2020; Iskander, 2020). However, the analysis of the spatialisation of power from "below" officialdom as a ramification of the viral shock is rare in the literature.

The stability theories of international relations often perceive a statist hegemon as a paramount authority that holds the centre together in the world order characterised by anarchy (Kindleberger, 1981; Webb &Krasner, 1989). Nevertheless, the influence asserted by the world's major powers and non-state actors, as well as the weaknesses of state institutions in regions of sub-Saharan Africa, undermines any conception of a statist regional hegemon responsible for regional stability. It is on this note that this chapter advances the literature by focusing on non-state mobile power structures within the regional security architecture in West Africa. This phenomenon is appraised in the laboratory of the ecological shock brought about by the COVID-19 pandemic in the region. Thus, this chapter complements the scientific literature by examining regional security entanglement from "below" in line with the biopolitics and geopolitics of public health in West Africa beyond the "top-down" approach popular in the literature.

DOI: 10.4324/9781003415121-5

Conceptual clarifications

The term "entanglement" points to the inseparability of matters in line with the logic of quantum physics (Barad, 2007; Verlie, 2017). In this vein, the interaction of matters forecloses the objectification of boundaries in physical existence. Beyond being an "interweaving" of "complicated" networks, entanglement implies an absence of "independent existence" (Barad,2007). On the other hand, geopolitics is a product of human geography. It is concerned with the systematic analysis of the uniqueness and relationship of places (Flint, 2006). It focuses on the uniqueness of places as conditioned by environmental and social factors with an emphasis on the spatial pattern of diverse livelihood. In this way, the geopolitics of health in the COVID-19 era measures the peculiar pattern and effect of health interventions in tandem with the socio-spatial location in the pluralistic global existence.

The spatial pattern of society illuminates its politics and power relations. In this vein, geopolitics, more than state actors, scramble for territories, including the quest by non-state actors to control territories amidst competition – a phenomenon that implies the multiple practices and representations of varied territories in place and space (Flint, 2006). This phenomenon is often revealed in a time of eco-social shock such as a pandemic when health interventions and local responses found expression in the pre-existing interactive ecological and social relations – an objectification of the biopolitics and geopolitics of health.

Pandemics are matters of global security. As observed by Stefan and Gemma (2019: 5), security is an "intensely reactional phenomenon that does not exist before, nor independently of, its intra-action with other agencies". Security and power are mutually connected. Scientific advancement influences security configuration due to its impact on the power structure in the global system. For instance, the development of nuclear weapons following World War II (1939–1945) was fundamental to the structuring of new world order (Falk, 1977). On the other hand, the pattern of global virus morbidity, whether engendered by natural causes or deliberately produced by bioterrorism, impacts the world differently due to divergent patterns of responses as informed by local peculiarities and resources in the global world system. The way scientific knowledge is marshalled to abate or prolong such spread impacts international security and the global structure of power.

Science may be seen as "separate from . . . [but] . . . subordinate to, the overriding security logics of anarchy" (Stefan &Gemma, 2019: 6). In this way, science is a lame world in itself but subject to the social instrumentalisation of knowledge. However, it has been noted that security and science like other elements of the planetary ecology are ontologically inseparable fields due to their mutually entangled networks (Barad, 2007; Stefan &Gemma, 2019). Scientific knowledge decodes the DNA of nature, including the physical and the biological, thereby ascribing control and power to knowledge. Insecurity is a product of ignorance and the inability to control the knowledge of nature and culture. Thus, security is guarded by an exercise of power that resides in knowledge. In essence, science and the social phenomenon interact in the production of cycles of power in society.

The ideas of health and security are mutually entangled. Security is a complex concept due to its multifarious manifestations as human, health, economic, social, food, national, and international securities. In harmonising the security complex, Wolfers (1952) noted that security is the "absence of threats to acquired values" – "a low probability of damage to acquire values". As observed by Baldwin (1997: 13), "security in its most general sense can be defined in terms of two specifications: 'security for whom' and 'security for which value'". The complexity of the concept of security produces "ambiguity" and "confusion". This is particularly true in the conceptualisation of health security (Aldis, 2008). The interconnectivity of economic and health security implies that without the duo, "it might be difficult for personal, political, community and food security to be ensured in a state" (Umukoro, 2020: 20). This affirms Faleye's (2021) position that global health history is an integrative history traversing socio-economic, political, international, and cross-border relations in an entangled global world system.

In harmonising the multi-faceted pattern of security, the United Nations observed the synergy provided by the concept of human security as total security, implying the security of both individuals, groups of people, and the state (UNDP, 1994). The concept of human security shows the inalienability of the social element of security despite the reality of preferentiality in security architecture. While security is valued by different actors, it cannot exist in isolation, as other contending needs are "sacrificed" in the pursuit of security. Therefore, the relevance of security on the scale of preference is simultaneously determined by the relativity of other existential threats of non-security concern. Thus, health security is contextualised here as security for all human beings in line with the absence of deadly threats to human biological well-being irrespective of the geographical location and social identity. This does not put into cognisance the security from war and socioeconomic threats. It is against this background that health security emerges on top of state, regional, and global security agendas in a time of public health crisis such as the COVID-19 pandemic. Again, the role of science in resolving the biological and ecological dilemma is re-invoked in line with the universality of scientific enquiry. This has led to the adoption of transnational principles of disease abatement and common health interventions of quarantine and movement restrictions without cognition for local peculiarities. Consequently, the interconnectivity of the web of security is brought to the fore by the peculiar local responses to health interventions that reinforce the emergency of other dimensions of security in West Africa – affirming the regional security entanglement.

The geopolitics of diseases such as the COVID-19 pandemic reveals the vulnerabilities present in the "uneven" spread and responses to a global viral outbreak. This has metamorphosed into "uneven geographies" of health that found expression in "uneven" health interventions and local responses to a pandemic that respects no state boundary (Pulignano &Marà, 2020). The spatialisation of power in pandemic

governance manifests in the peculiarity of the place, identity, pattern of disease aeti-
ology, health interventions, and local responses. Hence, infectious disease processes
present a web of socio-economic, political, transnational, and cross-border dynamics
with implications for public health.

In the strategic management of infectious disease outbreaks, the notion of
movement restrictions refers to every measure adopted to control human mobility through state power. Movement restriction as used here refers to public health
measures, including cordon sanitaire and quarantine, deployed to isolate COVID-19
foci. Cordon sanitaire is an impersonal version of quarantine that isolates perceived
infected spaces rather than persons. Unlike quarantine, which depends on the clinical manifestation of disease in a stipulated time, such as 14 days, for the isolation of
exposed persons is adjudged to be terminal in the coronavirus cycle, cordon sanitaire
isolates a space based on the socio-political perception of an existential threat of disease outbreak (Iskander, 2020). Historians and political philosophers have long identified a pattern of governmental control of people and space by social mapping of the
geography of contagion in the age of empire – the biopolitics of health (Bashford,
2004). Armstrong (1993) observed the making of public health spaces through the
fabrication of identity. In this vein, movement restrictions such as cordon sanitaire
as a measure of containing "diseased", "dirty", or "polluted" spaces operationalise
"rules of hygiene", "like religious interdictions", "a process of keeping separate" the
other (Armstrong 1993: 393). This spatialisation of power is obvious in the "structures and infrastructures for the control and management of past colonial empires
and current global firms and markets" (Sassen, 2001: 13). Social stratification in society creates a scale of preference for resource distribution, especially in a time of social
shock such as infectious disease spread which manifests in the public health policy
of movement restrictions, cordon sanitaire, and lockdowns as forms of bordering in
society. This is a governmental bordering of life or death through the mechanism of
public health interventions.

The power distribution in the past and present societies creates unequal places
and spaces by invoking the bordering of human relations with implications for human security. Hence, borders are conceived herein as legal limits delineated not
only at the state boundaries but also by regulations including public health policies
that partition identity within the state. However, local responses to these bordering
structures produce security ramifications that tilt the health security phenomenon
into other security emergencies, especially in a West African region battling with
the hellfire of glocal insurgency.

This brings to the fore the inseparability of the epidemiological shock from international relations and security. In the context of the discourse of power in the
making of spaces of health and security, this chapter assesses how movement restrictions such as cordon sanitaire and lockdowns were used to restrict or consolidate
class access to space, place, and resources. Here, the extant literature is robustly built
on the top-down approach to the spatialisation of power. In advancing this discourse, the complex implications and ramifications of the COVID-19 intervention

as exemplified by the regional security entanglement with the spatialisation of power from "below" in West Africa is offered as a complement to the extant literature on the geopolitics and biopolitics of health.

Reframing COVID-19 interventions: transnational responses and security entanglement in West Africa

The outbreak of the COVID-19 pandemic in Wuhan was officially reported by China on 31 December 2019. Subsequently, person-to-person and transnational spread of the infection was reported beyond China in Australasia, Asia, Europe, and North America (Phelan et al., 2020). The first case of the virus in Africa was recorded in Egypt on 14 February 2020 due to an international travel network connecting the continent with China (Loembé et al., 2020). In West Africa, the first case was reported in Nigeria on 27 February 2020 (Nigerian Center for Disease Control – NCDC, 2020). Subsequently, cases were recorded in other West African countries (Tchole et al., 2020). Considering the spread of the virus along with transportation infrastructure and social networks, the West African countries followed the historical path of implementing the public health measure of movement restrictions to delay the spread of the novel coronavirus (WHO, 2021a). By 25 June 2021, the World Health Organization reported total fatalities of 482 in Mauritania, 110 in Liberia, 329 in Ivory Coast, 2118 in Nigeria, 193 in Niger, 168 in Burkina Faso, 128 in Togo, 104 in Benin, 794 in Ghana, 87 in Sierra Leone, 168 in Guinea, 525 in Mali, 1159 in Senegal, and 69 deaths in Guinea Bissau (WHO, 2021b).

The state boundaries in West Africa are colonially determined. Even though cultural boundaries existed in pre-colonial West Africa, the colonial and post-colonial boundaries bifurcate the cultural areas in the region (Asiwaju, 2010; Miles, 1994). The influence of the cultural network that transcends these artificial boundaries is already over-flogged in the literature (Miles, 1994; Walter et al., 2015; Faleye, 2016, 2020). Nevertheless, the boundaries are recognised as legal limits and territorial delineations of the modern state with distinct colonial orientations. The management of borders and borderlands is central to any pandemic spread and control. Hence, a pandemic is a potent security issue in the international system. It is therefore not surprising that the legality of borderlines is often emphasised in a time of transnational pathogenic threat. Consequently, the COVID-19 pandemic is an important case in point where the viral spread stimulated international responses in line with travel bans and border closure. In this case, border closure represents a wider national form of cordon sanitaire invoked against international threats in the national interest.

Transnational infectious disease spread calls for international socio-economic and political responses with implications for the evolution of the governance architecture of the global world system. In this vein, the COVID-19 pandemic is a major test for the Western-centric liberal democratic order and its stranglehold on global politics (Samaddar, 2020). In a world facing a rising wave of nationalism, terrorism, xenophobia, and racism, the outbreak of the COVID-19 pandemic complicates the already fragile global world system. The invocation of national interest has found expression in the construction of boundaries of otherness in resource distribution and knowledge. These have manifested in the socio-scientific ideas of quarantines, cordon sanitaire, and lockdowns. These control measures have been rooted in the geopolitics of social denial which restricted vulnerable people's access to movement, food, medicine, and education in the face of governmental inefficiency. Indeed, the regional response to the pandemic spread amidst poor and weakly footed state institutions was marked by unprecedented regional, national, and human security issues in West Africa.

The pandemic illustrates how world cities such as Wuhan, Beijing, and New York showcase the spatialisation of power in nodes of global production and distribution networks. The challenge of this global frame of power has been brought to the fore by the rapid distribution of the coronavirus into the various connecting nerves of this global socio-economic network. The global public health approach to the COVID-19 spread showcases a policy of death in which the "hot spots were isolated" in line with the "boundary drawing strategy to arbitrate the number of deaths" (Samaddar, 2020: 6). In a globalising world reliant on the functionality of interconnected trade and transportation networks, border restrictions have impacted the global economy. The crisis of movement restrictions amidst a rising rocket of nationalism around the world has had a serious degrading impact on migrants. Beyond migrants, bordering could take effect from non-state impulses within the national territory. As noted by Agbiboa (2020), in the face of the pandemic, the Boko Haram barricade of supply chain networks was a bordering humanitarian aid in the Lake Chad region of West Africa.

The rapidity of human entanglement and infectious disease globalisation has led to the reinforcement of a nationalist agenda and bordering of relations in public policy. This is a contradiction of the globalisation and nationalism enhanced by the COVID-19 pandemic. For instance, the strengthening of nationalist movements in the wake of the viral spread has been noted in countries such as Qatar, the United States, and China, amongst others (Iskander, 2020). In West Africa, movement restrictions were implemented to terminate the pathogenic transmission. This had socio-economic implications concerning productivity in farming, trading, and the service sector which translated to food insecurity (Bisson & Hambleton, 2020). Despite the artificial nature and porousness of the colonially determined borders in Africa, public health regulations in the COVID-19 era have followed the closed border framework. Nevertheless, informal flows continued across these boundaries with implications for regional security and the power architecture of the region.

Despite its biological posture, COVID-19 and its attendant public health intervention influenced and implemented through state power unveil a politics of disease and health with a geopolitical complexion. The COVID-19 interventions in West Africa reveal the dynamism of public health policies as conduits for the negotiation of power in the region. This circumstance brings to the fore the glocality of human entanglement. In this vein, the closure of many businesses, truncation of value chains, scarcity of goods, high-mark inflation, massive job loss, high cost of living, and low standard of living impacted regional security in West Africa. The high unemployment level and the dominance of the informal sector in the regional economy made the lockdown procedures a death trap. Indeed, local testimonies affirm that many people starved in the confine of their homes with little or no governmental intervention during the lockdowns in Nigeria. This reality is confirmed by media reports by investigative journalists. As an extract from an interview survey published by DW puts it:

> I have to struggle in the crowd because there is no food at home and I need to get food for my daughter, my mum, my sister and her children, said Folashade Samuel, a Lagos slum dweller. Samuel is among a growing number of desperate Nigerians who risk stampedes to collect free food supplies. The single mother and her sister carry their babies on their backs to get more, but sometimes have to come home empty-handed. "We were scrambling for food when my sister with a young baby on her back was pushed away, and she had to give up," Samuel said. "The situation is a very, very tough. It is very dangerous to scramble for food because you can fall and get trampled on".
>
> *(DW, 2020)*

The challenge of food security is a symptom of African underdevelopment. This issue is central to the stability of the continent in the context of disease control and social conflicts. Indeed, at the root of Africa's disease burden such as Lassa fever and Ebola is the ecological intrusion into animal spaces with attendant eco-social reactions through disease outbreaks. In addition, social conflict over resource distribution is often a fallout from food insecurity. This is the case with the series of farmers-herders conflicts arising from nomadic pastoralism and encroachment into farmlands and grazing routes. Moreover, while food insecurity is not a legal excuse for criminality, the failure of African states to address issues of social services witnessed local responses through terrorism, banditry, and armed robbery. These conditions existed before the outbreak of COVID-19 in Africa. Thus, public health measures of movement restrictions adapted to control the viral spread threatened the already fragile security architecture, the infrastructure of food production, and supply.

In tackling the deepened food security challenges occasioned by COVID-19, the regional institutional intervention includes the protection of agriculture as an essential activity in the continent by the African Union (AU) and the Food and Agricultural Organization (FAO). For instance, in West Africa, the impact of this policy intervention was very obvious. In Nigeria, it has been noted that the movement restrictions have little impact on wage earners and farming activities but serious implications in the context of food security on families that are dependent on non-agricultural livelihoods (Amare et al., 2021). It is important to add that many wage earners experienced salary cuts, while others, unfortunately, lost their jobs – a situation which undermined the food security of many households. Mbatha et al. (2021) noted the breakdown of informal networks of food supply and distribution chains and the subsequent difficulties faced by the poor in this regard. The South African government, with one of the most serious COVID-19 disease burdens in Africa, responded to panic buying and the food shortages through the intervention of the National Policy on Food and Nutritional Security. However, inadequate storage facilities imply the distribution of spoilt food in South Africa, with medical consequences. These challenges call for policies that prioritise internal production within Africa rather than over-reliance on the global food supply chain.

Public health interventions showcase the power structure of society (Faleye et al., 2023). Considering the poor regional public health emergency preparedness, the pandemic created the basis for foreign financial aid as well as emergency re-allocation of existing funds to health interventions in West Africa. Movement restrictions, cordon sanitaire, and lockdowns provided the need for unusual aid whose medium of distribution is inherently lacking in accountability. At the centre of health, intervention is the issue of social justice. The outbreak of the coronavirus and the ensuing movement restrictions necessitated the need for government engagement with the people in the area of social justice. This is particularly important, since countering the pandemic requires the provision of social security. This is challenging considering the decadence of social services in countries of the region owing to poor governance over the years.

As observed by Stickle and Felson (2020), the health intervention measures involving movement restrictions around the world had reduced daily travels and commercial routines, as many people began to work from home except for essential workers. The attendant change in people's livelihood brought about by public health ordinance is believed to have reduced the occurrence of crime around the world. However, the pandemic pathology and the multiplicity of public health interventions around the world produce distinct local responses. For instance, it has been observed that the pandemic led to internal security issues in Nigeria (Okolie-Osemene, 2021). The sudden spread of coronavirus disease to West Africa impacted the security architecture, as the region was battling an insurgency. Before the public health restrictions, the country faced internal security challenges such as armed robbery, banditry, and militancy. The outbreak led to the diversion of the existing security architecture to the enforcement of lockdowns and contact tracing.

A cross-border informal network is at the centre of West African socio-economic and political architecture (Asiwaju, 2001, 2010; Nugent, 2008; Walther et al., 2015; Faleye, 2016, 2020). The challenges of poor social services before the outbreak of COVID-19 complicated the long-standing problem of a government deficit in West Africa. The implication was the entrenchment of alternative non-state regional political articulations with security implications in the region. While the closed border approach restricted activities in the formal sector, it created spaces of vacuum and reinforced alternative power networks of mobile culture in under-governed spaces such as forest areas that were under serious ethnocultural contentions before the COVID-19 outbreak. The unofficial regional entanglement manifested in contradictions of both movement restriction and acceleration of intra-regional migration in the COVID-19 era. The phenomenon reveals the regional security entanglement through the ramifications of public health policies and its implication for the restructuring of spaces of power in West Africa. As observed by the mayor of Arlit in the Republic of Niger (a transit corridor in West Africa), Abderahmane Maouli, "Despite the border closure, we see that movements are continuing: People travel through minor routes to avoid border controls and reach Arlit without going through the quarantine, and this is a major public health issue for our community" (Maouli quoted in Zandonini, 2020). Moreover, this scenario was noted by the International Organisation for Migration's (IOM's) chief of mission in Niger, Barbara Rijks, thus: "While the borders are officially closed, we still see migrants arriving in Niger from neighbouring countries that need to complete 14 days of mandatory quarantine" (IOM, 2020).

An important attribute of a state is territoriality (Agnew, 2005). The status of state power is revealed by the extent to which a state could mobilise its security apparatus in the enforcement of socio-spatial legal limits within its territory. This does not necessarily imply the absence of militia-governed spaces in a state, but could include the state's ability to engage in diplomatic engagement with such spaces to reinforce peace and security (Jagadish, 2009). This proposes a complexity of a state mechanism in reinforcing its legal boundaries and human security not only through force but also interactive entanglement with non-state actors. Indeed, in world political history, the contestation of the central authority is often nurtured at the fringes of state territory. Nevertheless, borders and borderlands, with their fluidity, become neutral as non-state political agitations and manoeuvrings are nourished by the weakness of central authorities rather than the spatial spaces between and within states (Olaniyan et al., 2021). It is therefore obvious that the spatialisation of power from the top or down of a political structure hinges on the nature of state security. It is on this note that the changing configuration of the power structure and regional entanglement in West Africa in the COVID-19 era is a direct reflection of the transformational role of how actors responded to the health interventions in the aftermath of the public health shock in the region. Thus, the timeline of public health measures such as movement restrictions could be seen as an incubation period, setting into place the reconfiguration of governance in West African mobile and ungoverned spaces.

Studies have noted the endurance of militarism and terrorism despite the horror of the public health shock as the pandemic presents conduits of opportunities for non-state militias. The exploitation of pandemic fear through conspiracy theories and propaganda orchestrated by militia groups is no longer news. For instance, the outbreak witnessed militia propaganda as Sunni jihadists reportedly emphasised that the viral outbreak was a product of anti-Islamic elements, while al-Qaeda and ISIS argue it is a manifestation of Allah's wrath against a corrupt capitalist world (Bloom, 2020; Kruglanski et al., 2020; Ackerman &Peterson, 2020). The exploitation of security gaps as a result of the overwhelming pressure of COVID-19 on social services impacted militia operations. Scholars have forecasted the likelihood of the pandemic shock in transforming militia operations subject to the "levels of disruption and official control in the location where the terrorists are operating", thereby presenting militias contesting state power with "opportunities for expanding, or at least adapting, their activities, both violent and otherwise, and in certain circumstances might even act as a stimulus to action". Moreover, it has been argued that the pandemic disruptions – loss of lives, jobs, and livelihood – could stimulate psychological challenges and make vulnerable people susceptible to radicalisation (Ackerman &Peterson, 2020: 61–62). The governmental intervention during the lockdown in countries such as Nigeria reveals the spatialisation of power from "above" that tilts the distribution of state resources in the interest of the political elite class. The widespread corruption and the reported diversion of aid into the possession of the political elites widened the existing social landscape of inequality. The implication was a local response that found solace in a pre-existing alternative stream of power that thrives in under-governed spaces and regional criminality.

The instrumentality of public health measures of movement restrictions is cogent in expanding the frontier of non-state power in the regional hotbed of insurgency – Nigeria. In a region where land resources are fiercely contested between sedentary and nomadic groups, movement restrictions imply temporary displacement and the creation of a spatial vacuum. Thus, the ability to negotiate restrictive public health regulations across state boundaries by mobile cultures is instrumental to the spatialisation of power from below in the region. The distraction created by the COVID-19 pandemic and the consequent deployment of security forces to enforce public health ordinances witnessed the aggravation of Boko Haram attacks in the Nigerian northeast. Moreover, Campbell (2020) observed that amid the public health crisis the militia group operated freely – launching attacks and offering social services in the borderlands of Nigeria and Niger.

In West Africa, violent conflicts involving militia groups straddling state boundaries have led to the deaths of many people in the region (Walther &Miles, 2018; Trémolières et al., 2020). In January 2020, before the COVID-19 lockdown, Mohamed Ibn Chambas, the United Nations Special Representative and Head of the UN Office for West Africa and the Sahel (UNOWAS) observed that the "region has experienced a devastating surge in terrorist attacks against civilian and military targets". This is a case of rapidly rising fatalities accruing from political violence in West Africa, if we take into consideration the estimated 770 people killed in 2016 compared to about 4,000 murders committed in the trio of Mali, Burkina Faso, and Niger in 2019 with a geographic spread shifting eastwards from "Mali to Burkina-Faso and increasingly threatening West African coastal states" (United Nations, 2020). Beyond the insurgencies in the region, a significant proportion of these violent attacks is a product of cross-border pastoral nomadic banditry. The end of the lockdown confirmed Chambas's fear of the spread of the crisis to the West African coastal states as Nigeria was besieged by unprecedented banditry and kidnapping afforded by spaces governed by cross-border mobile bandits. For instance, an estimated 4,556 people were murdered in violent attacks, kidnappings, and banditry in Nigeria in 2020 compared to the 3,188 deaths recorded in 2019 (Global Rights, 2021; Adesomoju, 2021). The first quarter of 2021 marked the violent murder of 1,603 people with an estimated 1,774 people kidnapped in Nigeria due to the expanding activities of Islamic State West Africa Province, Boko-Haram, and bandit gangs in the country (Kabir, 2021).

In West Africa, the contradiction of public health measures and regional reality found expression in the dispersal of militia groups into spaces of the vacuum created by the health intervention. There are reports of north-south migration in which terrorists and bandit strong-holds in the Sahel dispersed towards the coastal settlements of West Africa, especially in Nigeria, where Boko-Haram's presence and banditry became emboldened in the savanna and kidnapping intensified at the coast in the aftermath of the lockdown measures. Indeed, this implies a socio-spatial spread of militia activities during the COVID-19 lockdown in West Africa. The lockdown witnessed the re-deployment of the military machinery, from counterterrorism operations to the enforcement of the quarantine ordinance. It marked an abrupt reduction in international security coalitions against terrorism. Thus, the lockdown measures opened up ungoverned spaces such as inter-state and inter-region frontiers and forests to militia flow and occupation. This created the foundation for the terrorist onslaught that spread beyond the Lake Chad region to most parts of Nigeria in the form of banditry involving kidnapping for ransom, human organ harvesting, and rape. It is not surprising therefore that the Lake Chad basin network of terror involving the chains of attacks by the Islamic State of West Africa, Boko-Haram, nomadic pastoral militias, and bandits has skyrocketed in the post–COVID-19 lockdown in terms of violence perpetrated against unarmed civilian and military targets.

The COVID-19 disruptions found expression in the dislocation of police and military operations as well as the degrading of governmental institutions and the important role of the private sector in stabilising a weakened economy. Moreover, the excesses of police operatives in enforcing the lockdown measures and the resultant civil protest (End-SAS) marking the dissolution of the special unit such as the Special Anti-robbery Squad in the Nigerian police created a vacuum in civil policing and thereby strengthening the stronghold of militia groups in their mobile abode. It is within these diverse local responses to COVID-19 that the rising militarisation of West Africa and Nigeria in particular could be explained in the COVID-19 era. The COVID-19 fatalities in West Africa are particularly low compared to other regions of the world. This low incidence of the viral spread cannot be attributed to the lockdown, as the lockdown never affected social distancing, since parties and the mingling of people in living quarters located in areas with poor infrastructure, especially in cities such as Lagos, lingered on. In addition, informal movement within the state and across borders in West African countries such as Nigeria and Niger thrived amidst the health interventions. Indeed, the COVID-19 projects global health entangled with peculiar regional security frameworks – a glocality of entangled security reality.

Concluding remarks

The COVID-19 pandemic affirms the entanglement of nature and cultures in the global world system. This chapter reveals the complexity of the entanglement of the security agenda as the public health interventions in line with the ideas of health security impacted other forms of security such as economic security, state security, and human security in West Africa. It unveils the spatialisation of power from below during a public health crisis as rare in the literature on the biopolitics and geopolitics of health. It examines how policy choices in respect of health security opened up new conduits of opportunities for militia growth in ungoverned areas from the Sahel to the coast of West Africa. The phenomenon unveils a peculiarity of security entanglement in West Africa.

Furthermore, the coronavirus outbreak presented West Africa with peculiar choices and opportunities to outrun other regions and offset its economic deficits by implementing peculiar public health measures adaptable to its security and economic predicaments or follow the band-wagon of the Anglo-European public health bordering initiatives as an extension of the neo-colonial global empire lacking local initiatives and relegated to the dungeon of the global economy and political architecture. Unfortunately, West Africa, and Nigeria in particular, choose the latter, thereby collapsing its fragile regional security infrastructure and degrading the economy in exchange for theoretical Eurocentric health security that lacks an understanding of the African environment. Nigeria is the heartbeat of West Africa, hence its policy choices impact migration and cross-border flows with implications for human security in the region. The local and regional responses to the Nigerian COVID-19 intervention marked an unprecedented collapse of the state apparatus in the country, with terrorist, bandits, and militia groups in the region strategically spread across the country and boldly engaging Nigerian security agencies and civilians. This is the outcome of the complex interactions between health security, state security, and the implications for human security in an entangled regional livelihood and pluralistic global coexistence.

References

Ackerman, G. and Peterson, H. 2020. Terrorism and COVID-19. *Perspectives on Terrorism*, 14(3): 59–73.

Adesomoju, A. 2021. 4,556 persons killed in violent attacks, kidnappings, clashes in 2020 – Report. *Premium Times*, February 22. www.premiumtimesng.com/news/headlines/444634-4556-persons-killed-in-violent-attacks-kidnappings-clashes-in-2020-report.html

Agbiboa, D. E. 2020. COVID-19, Boko Haram and the pursuit of survival: A battle of lives against livelihoods. *City & Society*, 32(2): 1–14. https://doi.org/10.1111/CISO.12307

Agnew, J. 2005. Sovereignty regimes: Territoriality and state authority in contemporary world politics. *Annals of the Association of American Geographers*, 95(2): 437–461.

Aldis, W. 2008. Health security as a public health concept: A critical analysis. *Health Policy and Planning*, 23: 369–375.

Amare, M., Abay, K.A., Tiberti, L. and Chamberlin, J. 2021. COVID-19 and food security: Panel data evidence from Nigeria. *Food Policy*, 101. https://doi.org/10.1016/j.foodpol.2021.102099

Armstrong, D. 1993. Public health spaces and the fabrication of identity. *Sociology*, 27(3): 393–410.

Asiwaju, A. I. 2001. The implementation of ECOWAS treaty and protocols: The role of workers and civil society in the context of a comparison with the history of the European Union. *Lagos Historical Review*, 1: 45–58.

Asiwaju, A. I. 2010. Cross-border initiatives and regional integration in West Africa: The Nigerian experience. In *Nation-States and the Challenges of Regional Integration in West Africa: The Case of Nigeria*, edited by Akinyeye Eniola, pp. 137–148. Paris: Karthala.

Baldwin, D. A. 1997. The concept of security. *Review of International Studies*, 23: 5–26.

Barad, K. 2007. *Meeting the Universe Halfway: Quantum Physics and the Entanglement of Matter and Meaning*. Durham: Duke University Press.

Bashford, A. 2004. *Imperial Hygiene: A Critical History of Colonialism, Nationalism and Public Health*. Basingstoke: Palgrave Macmillan.

Bisson, L. and Hambleton, T. 2020. COVID-19 Impact on West African Value Chains. In *CRU Policy Brief*. Clingendael: Netherlands Institute of International Relations.

Bloom, M. 2020. How terrorist groups will try to capitalize on the Coronavirus crisis. *Just Security*, April 3. www.justsecurity.org/69508/how-terrorist-groups-will-tryto-capitalize-on-the-coronavirus-crisis/

Campbell, J. 2020. Beyond the pandemic, boko haram looms large in Nigeria. *Council on Foreign Relations*. www.jstor.org/stable/resrep29819

DW. 2020. *Severe Hunger Threatens Africa during COVID-19 Lockdowns*, 22 April. www.dw.com/en/severe-hunger-threatens-africa-during-covid-19-lockdowns/a-53212565

Faleye, O. A. 2016. Regional integration from 'below' in West Africa: A study of transboundary town-twinning of Idiroko (Nigeria) and Igolo (Benin). *Regions & Cohesion*, 6(3): 1–18.

Faleye, O. A. 2020. Unveiling the Afro-European common geo-cultural space. In *Expanding Boundaries: Borders, Mobilities and the Future of Europe-Africa Relations*, edited by J. P. Laine, Inocent Moyo and Christopher Changwe Nshimbi. London: Routledge.

Faleye, O. A. 2021. Explaining disease: A chapter in Nigerian historiography. *Social Evolution & History*, 20(1): 94–113. https://doi.org/10.30884/she/2021.01.04.

Faleye, O. A., Akande, T. M. and Moyo, I. 2023. *Public Health in Postcolonial Africa: The Social and Political Determinants of Health*. London: Routledge.

Falk, R. 1977. Nuclear weapons proliferation as a world order problem. *International Security*, 1(3): 79–93.

Flint, C. 2006. *Introduction to Geopolitics*. London: Routledge.

Global Rights. 2021. *Mass Atrocities Report: 2020*, 28 May. https://www.globalrights.org/ng/wp-content/uploads/2021/02/Mass-Atrocities-report-2020.pdf

Grundy-Wan, C. and Lin, S. 2020. COVID-19 geopolitics: Silence and erasure in Cambodia and Myanmar in times of pandemic. *Eurasian Geography and Economics*, 61: 493–510. https://doi.org/10.1080/15387216.2020.1780928

Harvey, D. 2020. *Anti-Capitalist Politics in the Time of COVID-19*. https://jacobinmag.com/2020/03/david-harvey-coronavirus-political-economydisruptions

International Organisation for Migration (IOM). 2020. *IOM Steps Up Response for Migrants Stranded in Niger Amidst COVID-19 Lockdown*. www.iom.int/news/iom-steps-response-migrants-stranded-niger-amidst-covid-19-lockdown

Iskander, N. 2020. Qatar, the Coronavirus, and Cordons Sanitaires, Migrant workers and the use of public health measures to define the nation. *Medical Anthropology Quarterly*, 34(4): 561–577.

Jagadish, V. 2009. Reconsidering American strategy in South Asia: Destroying terrorist sanctuaries in Pakistan's tribal areas. *Small Wars &Insurgencies*, 20(1): 36–65.

Kabir, A. 2021. 1,603 killed, 1,774 abducted in violent attacks across Nigeria in three months – Report. *Premium Times*, 17 May. www.premiumtimesng.com/news/headlines/461986-1603-killed-1774-abducted-in-violent-attacks-across-nigeria-in-three-months-report.html

Kindleberger, C. 1981. Dominance and leadership in the international economy: Exploitation, Public goods and free rides. *International Studies Quarterly*, 25(2): 242–254.

Kruglanski, A. W., Gunaratna, R., Ellenberg, M. and Speckhard, A. 2020. Terrorism in time of the pandemic: Exploiting mayhem. *Global Security: Health, Science and Policy*, 5(1): 121–132. https://doi.org/10.1080/23779497.2020.1832903

Loembé, M., Tshangela, A., Salyer, S. J., Varma, J. K., Ouma, A. E. O. and Nkengasong, J. N. 2020. COVID-19 in Africa: The spread and response. *Nature Medicine*, 26(7): 999–1003.

Mbatha, M. W., Ndimande, N. J. and Tembe, K. S. 2021. COVID-19 pandemic and food security in South Africa: The government's response. *African Renaissance*, 18(4): 305–317.

Memon, Z., Qureshi, S. and Memon, B. R. 2021. Assessing the role of quarantine and isolation as control strategies for COVID-19 outbreak: A case study. *Chaos, Solitons & Fractals*, 144. https://doi.org/10.1016/j.chaos.2021.110655

Miles, F. S. W. 1994. *Hausaland Divided: Colonialism and Independence in Nigeria and Niger*. New York: Cornell University Press.

Nigerian Center for Disease Control. 2020. *First Case of Corona Virus Disease Confirmed in Nigeria*, 28 February. https://ncdc.gov.ng/news/227/first-case-of-corona-virus-disease-confirmed-in-nigeria

Nugent, P. 2008. Not so much boom towns as trickle towns: A comparison of two West African Border Towns; Kpetoe (Ghana) and Darsilami (Gambia). In *Essays in Honour of Anthony Asiwaju*, edited by Y. Akinyeye, pp. 84–105. Imeko: Africa Regional Institute.

Okolie-Osemene, J. 2021. Nigeria's security governance dilemmas during the COVID-19 crisis. *Politikon*, 48(2): 260–277. https://doi.org/10.1080/02589346.2021.1913802

Olaniyan, R. A., Faleye, O. A. and Moyo, I. (eds.). 2021. *Transborder Pastoral Nomadism and Human Security in Africa: Focus on West Africa*. London: Routledge.

Phelan, A., Gotz, R. and Gostin, L. O. 2020. The novel coronavirus originating in Wuhan, China: Challenges for global health governance. *JAMA*, 323(8): 709–710.

Pulignano, V. and Marà, C. 2020. *The Coronavirus, Social Bonds and the 'Crisis Society'*. www.socialeurope.eu/the-coronavirussocial-bonds-and-the-crisis-society

Samaddar, R. (ed.). 2020. *Borders of an Epidemic: COVID-19 and Migrant Workers*. Kolkata: Mahanirban Calcutta Research Group.

Sassen, S. 2001. *Globalization and Its Discontents*. New York: The New Press.

Stefan, E. and Gemma, B. 2019. Entangled security: Science, Co-production and intra-active in security. *European Journal of International Security*, 4(2): 123–141 (Sussex Research Online). http://sro.sussex.ac.uk/id/eprint/81292/

Stickle B. and Felson, M. 2020. Crime rates in a pandemic: The largest criminological experiment in history. *American Journal of Criminal Justice*, 45: 525–536. https://doi.org/10.1007/s12103-020-09546-0

Tchole, A. I. M., Li, Z., Wei, J., Ye, R., Wang, W., Du, W., Wang, H., Yin, C., Ji, X., Xue, F., Maman, A., Zhao, L. and Cao, W. 2020. Epidemic and control of COVID-19 in Niger: Quantitative analyses in a least developed country. *Journal of Global Health*, 20(2). https://doi.org/10.7189/jogh.10.020513

Trémolières, M., Walther, O. and Radil, S. (eds.). 2020. *The Geography of Conflict in North and West Africa*. Paris: OECD.

Umukoro, N. 2020. Corona virus disease outbreak and human security in Africa. *Journal of Peacebuilding and Development*, 16(2): 254–258.

UNDP. 1994. *Human Development Report*. Oxford: Oxford University Press.

United Nations. 2020. Unprecedented terrorist violence in West Africa, Sahel region. *Peace and Security*, 8 January. https://news.un.org/en/story/2020/01/1054981

Van Dorn, A., Cooney, R. E. and Sabin, M. L. 2020. COVID-19 Exacerbating inequalities in the US. *The Lancet*, 395: 1243–1244. https://doi.org/10.1016/S0140-6736(20)30893-X

Verlie, B. 2017. Rethinking climate education: Climate as entanglement. *Educational Studies*, 53(6): 560–572. https://doi.org/10.1080/00131946.2017.1357555

Walther, O.J., Howard, A.M. and Retaille, D. 2015. West African spatial patterns of economic activities: Combining the 'spatial factor' and 'mobile space' approaches. *African Studies*, 74(3): 346–365.

Walther, O. and Miles, W. (eds.). 2018. *African Border Disorders. Addressing Transnational Extremist Organizations*. London: Routledge.

Webb, M. C. and Krasner, S. D. 1989. Hegemonic stability theory: An empirical assessment. *Review of International Studies*, 15(2): 183–198.

WHO. 2021a. *COVID-19 Report*, 3 June. https://covid19.who.int/region/afro/country/ne

WHO. 2021b. *WHO Coronavirus (COVID-19) Dashboard*, 25 June. https://covid19.who.int/

Wolfers, A. 1952. National security as an ambiguous symbol. *Political Science Quarterly*, 67(4): 481–502.

Zandonini, G. 2020. Hundreds of migrants stuck in Niger amid coronavirus pandemic. *Aljazeera News*, 9 April. www.aljazeera.com/news/2020/4/9/hundreds-of-migrants-stuck-in-niger-amid-coronavirus-pandemic

6

THE CONUNDRUM OF BALANCING BETWEEN COVID-19 POLICING AND HUMAN RIGHTS PROTECTION IN SOUTH AFRICA

A responsibility to protect perspective (R2P)

Patrick Dzimiri

Introduction and background

SARS-CoV- 2, commonly known as COVID-19, was declared a global pandemic on 11 March 2020 (WHO, 2020). The transnational dynamics of the pandemic were felt across the globe, having started in the city of Wuhan in China, and later spread across the globe. In South Africa, the first case of the virus was reported in Pietermaritzburg on 5 March 2020 when a South African national who had travelled to Europe showed signs of COVID-19 infection (South African Government Press Release, 2022; WHO, 2022; National Institute for Communicable Diseases, 2020). The pervasive manner in which the COVID-19 virus spreads compelled countries across the globe to adopt inward-looking policies by imposing national lockdowns to curb the spread of the virus (Mawarire, 2020). The period of national lockdowns epitomised an era of deglobalisation as countries desperately tried to save their citizens from contracting COVID-19 by closing their borders, ports of entry, and national airports. Restricting the free movement of people, compulsory wearing of face masks, and social distancing were among the prime measures embraced by countries to save lives, South Africa included.

In South Africa, a National Corona Virus Command Council (NCCC) was established to advise the government on the appropriate response to the pandemic. Every sector of human undertaking, from business, schools, and social life, was disrupted by successive national lockdown measures as the country battled the pandemic. COVID-19 responses adopted by the government of South Africa caused social and economic disruptions due to prolonged closures (Zwane, 2020). On the other hand, lives were lost as thousands of people capitulated to the virus. As of 5 July 2022, the pandemic claimed an estimated 101,815 lives and 3,995,400 cases of

DOI: 10.4324/9781003415121-6

COVID-19 infections have been recorded nationwide (WHO, 2022; South African Government Press Release, 2022).

On 23 June 2022 the government of South Africa (GoS), through the Ministry of Health, scrapped sections 16A and 16C of the National Health Act that regulates the containment of COVID-19. The repealed measures include the wearing of face masks, social distancing, restrictions on social gatherings, and screening at the ports of entry and public spaces (South African Government Press Release, 2022). While the relaxing of the regulations was based on the decline in COVID-19 infection rates, COVID-19–related deaths, and cases of hospitalisation (South African Government Press Release, 2022), the experience of mitigating the spread of the pandemic conspicuously exposed some cracks, particularly in the discharge of lockdown enforcement measures. The South African government (SA government) utilized the Emergency Services Act to contain the pandemic and swiftly moved to prioritise the deployment of security personnel to stop non-essential movement in the country. As will be articulated in the chapter, the draconian approach to lockdown enforcement premised on tacit military approaches had serious human rights repercussions. The "intended or unintended" human security costs of the military-enforced lockdowns raise questions regarding responsibility while protecting people from COVID-19. Fundamentally, the main questions guiding the analysis are (i) Could the GoS have rather evoked the R2P to authorise the delivery of security and protection against COVID-19 to non-consenting citizens? (ii) Would this have shifted the balance to human rights meriting protection?

The rest of the chapter is organised as follows: after this introduction, part two of the chapter discusses the R2P concept. Part three examines emergency disaster regulations introduced during the COVID-19 pandemic in South Africa and the anecdotal evidence of human rights violations. Part four concludes the chapter by scrutinising the military policing excesses during the lockdown period and analysing the state's response to the military's excesses. The analysis is framed in a human rights discourse that puts R2P as a critical driver in managing health pandemics.

Conceptual dimensions: the responsibility to protect principles

The responsibility to protect norm/principle, popularly known as R2P, was initially designed to protect civilians from crimes of a heinous nature (UN World Summit Outcome Document-, 2005; International Commission on Intervention and State Sovereignty, 2001). Considering wanton human rights violations of state-making, the R2P emphasises the primary responsibility of a state as the protection of its citizens. At the 2005 UN World Summit, the UN General Assembly (UNGA) Resolution 60/1.23 adopted the document on R2P but restricted its application to four specified crimes, namely, genocide, war crimes, ethnic cleansing, and crimes against humanity (UN World Summit, 2005). The targets to be protected and the perpetrators were clearly defined in this phrasing. Core to the R2P is the protection of citizens from life-threatening situations, and this chapter claims that the COVID-19 pandemic is one such public problem meriting its application. In situations of the state's manifest failure to protect its people, R2P usually benefits from oversight and often the intervention of external actors who assume the residual duty to protect (Jarvis, 2020; Smith, 2020; Evans, 2008; Thakur, 2016). Ironically, during a health pandemic like COVID-19, there is no external surveillance by others except for the localised media and independent defenders of democracy, and this leaves would-be victims in a vulnerable position. What is worse is the fact that given the global nature of COVID-19, every state/country was preoccupied with efforts to protect its own citizens, implying that there was little room to monitor what other countries were doing. Poignantly, the nature of the disease, and the way it spreads caused apprehension to the extent that policy decisions to combat the disease were often made in controversial circumstances.

The R2P concept resonates with the human security paradigm, as both give primacy to the protection of the population at risk and the security of people rather than territory (UNDP, 1994). Thus, emphasis is on the security of the people, rather than their territories (UNDP, 1994). Special emphasis is on people's physical safety, economic, and personal well-being; respect for their dignity and worth as human beings; and the protection of their human rights and fundamental freedoms (UNDP, 1994). This aligns with the United Nations Sustainable Development Goal 3 (UNSDG-3) regarding "good health and well-being" (UNSDG, 2015). Fittingly, the emphasis is on identifying threats to human lives and mitigating the threats before they degenerate into actual catastrophes. As the initial and one of the triad continuums of the R2P, the responsibility to prevent focuses on measures aimed at addressing catastrophes before they turn virulent. Despite the conceptual ambiguities and lack of consensus on the operational parameters of the R2P, the norm remains a useful framework to safeguard civilians from all avoidable harm (Jarvis, 2020; Smith, 2020). The lockdown measures, therefore, should be construed as constituting the internal (at national levels) prevention modalities developed by the governments to mitigate the spread of COVID-19. The extent to which the government of South Africa discharged its R2P mandate during the pandemic, however, remains a major bone of contention. Having construed the national lockdown measures within the ambience of the R2P norm, the next section provides a snapshot of the literature review on the human rights dimensions of COVID-19 lockdown measures across the globe.

Perspectives on COVID-19 and human rights protection

There is a paucity of literature analysing COVID-19 through the prism of the R2P norm. Scholars such as Jeiroudi (2021), Peak (2020), and Wambua (2020) attempted to streamline the R2P principle to cover the COVID-19 pandemic. Jeiroudi (2021) proposed an expanded version of R2P in addition to its conventional focus on war crimes and other crimes against humanity. The conventional focus of R2P proved to be limited because of its exclusive focus on human rights violations of a political making. The global nature of the pandemic meant that all states were more or less in similar situations and the concomitant lockdown responses were likely to put human rights at stake. The R2P concept could have been invoked to guide states' responses to the pandemic. COVID-19, therefore, exposed some inadequacies of the R2P doctrine's narrow-minded approach to human rights protection. Peak (2020) and Wambua (2020) submit that internally displaced people and refugees are vulnerable during the COVID-19 pandemic, hence the imperative to be protected by the state. Thus, the prevention framework of the R2P should be invoked for protecting such vulnerable groups. Peak (2020) proposes expanding the R2P or state's responsibilities to public health threats, which is beyond the conventional focus of the principle. The preceding view reasons well, considering the COVID-19 human rights violations experienced globally. Another concern has been raised to consider R2P when responding to COVID-19 specifically for repressive regimes whose conduct may threaten lives during the pandemic (Peak, 2020).

Reports on COVID-19–related human rights abuse across the globe are well-documented (Bekema, 2021; Herbert & Marquette, 2021; Cooper & Aitchison, 2021). Evidence shows that human rights abuses during national lockdowns have been a feature of both democratic and undemocratic governments. Herbert and Marquette (2021) acknowledge the role of state capacity and legitimacy in enforcing COVID-19 lockdown measures. They, however, underscore the importance of regime type in instituting and implementing COVID-19 responses. One aspect that came out strongly is that, globally, COVID-19–related human rights violations are more pronounced in autocratic regimes (Herbert & Marquette, 2021). One conspicuous aspect of lockdowns that has characterised national responses to the pandemic is what Gibson-Fall (2022: 2) describe as "blended civil-military responses" where the military is engaged in health-related matters. The phenomenon is attributed to the global-health security paradigm since the dawn of the century where militaries expand their mandate to include the provision of "medical, humanitarian and technical support" in times of pandemics (Gibson-Fall, 2022: 2). An argument about the health security nexus advanced by Davies (2008), Elbe (2006), and De Waal (2010) is that the reconceptualization of security to include diseases (epidemics and pandemics) as constituting non-violent and non-physical threats to humanity opened the floodgate for the military to play a pivotal role in fighting health-related human security threats. The expansive role of the military in health-related security threats such as Ebola, influenza, and Zika virus is recognised (Wenham & Farais, 2019; Harman & Wenham, 2018; Waterson & Kamradt-Scott, 2016). The Ebola outbreak in West Africa and Zika virus in China, for example, have seen military deployments to reinforce health practitioners (Gibson-Fall, 2021).

It turned out, however, that the military factor in lockdown enforcement in most countries fits the description of an "authoritarian turn" since several facets of human rights were restricted (Herbert & Marquette, 2021: 7). There are reports where political regimes in Zimbabwe and the Philippines, for example, used lockdown measures for consolidation and centralisation of power (Bueno de Mesquita et al., 2021; Herbert & Marquette, 2021; Williams et al., 2020). Similarly, Bekema (2021:

6) talks about the notion of "pandemics and punitive regulation" in the Philippines, citing the iron-fisted approach that trampled on citizens' human rights and freedoms. Such has been expressly described by Guterres (2021: 1) as constituting the "new pandemic of human rights abuses".

For many repressive regimes, the lockdown environment presented an opportune moment for punishing political rivals (Cooper & Aitchison, 2020; Williams et al., 2020). Comparable experiences in Hungary and India reveal an element of using complex emergencies for entrenching authoritarian governances (Cooper & Aitchison, 2020; Greer et al., 2020). The 2020 Human Rights Watch (HRW) report unmasked the challenges of homophobia, xenophobia, and discrimination in Poland during the lockdown period (HRW, 2020). In the case of China, there are reports of silencing descent as the media reported on appalling COVID-19 conditions in Wuhan Central Hospital (Li & Galea, 2020). Related developments are captured by Mawarire (2020), citing the criminalisation of reporting on COVID-19 in Zimbabwe, Eswatini, and Zambia. As a result, some measures instituted to curb the spread of COVID-19 infringed on the rights and freedoms of the citizens and departed completely from the democratic ethos (Mawarire, 2020).

At the global multi-lateral level, the United Nations Human Rights Commissioner, Mitchell Bachelet, unequivocally challenged that "emergency powers should not be a weapon government can wield to quash dissent, control population and even perpetuate their time in power" (Bachelet, 2020b: 1). Bachelet further condemned gross acts of shooting, abusing, and beating citizens for violating lockdown regulations (DefenseWeb, 2020). The World Health Organization (WHO, 2020) reinforces the inseparable relationship between COVID-19 and human rights protection by advocating human rights as a comprehensive package for mitigating COVID-19. Thus, the WHO director-general, Dr Tedros, implored countries to "strike a balance between protecting health, minimizing economic and social disruption and respecting human rights" (UNOHCHR, 2020: 1). Tedros further underscored that "emergency declarations based on the COVID-19 outbreak should not be used as a basis to target particular groups, minorities, or individuals" (UN News, 2020: 2). These assertions, therefore, make human rights protection key to effective COVID-19 responses.

The COVID-19 mitigation measures by the South African government

The transnational way in which COVID-19 unfolded required responsive governments and total commitment to the duty to protect their nationals. Pursuant to the confirmation of the first case of COVID-19, on 5 March 2020, the presidency established the NCCC, headed by Minister of Cooperative Governance and Traditional Affairs Nkosazana Dlamini-Zuma (Hosken, 2021; Heywood, 2020; Hofman & Madhi, 2020). The mandate was to guide the government in curbing the spread and dealing with the consequences of COVID-19 (Heywood, 2020).

Consistent with the R2P, the GoS invoked the Disaster Management Act to declare a state of national disaster on 27 March 2020 and implemented a national lockdown for 21 days (Heywood, 2020; Hofman & Madji, 2020; Levine & Manderson, 2020). The country was moved to Alert Level 5, characterised by massive restrictions on the free movement of people, closure of schools and businesses (except for those deemed essential services), banning the sale of alcohol and cigarettes, overall banning of public gatherings, compulsory wearing of face masks, and observing social distancing (South African Government Gazette, 2021; Hofman & Madhi, 2020). In a similar fashion, the inter-provincial movement had to be sanctioned by the government authorities and the national borders were partially closed while, international travels were restricted (Hofman & Madhi, 2020). Sections 201(2) (a) of the Constitution of the Republic of South Africa, 1996 and Section 18(1)(a) and Section 19 of the Republic of Defence Act, Act 42 of 2002 were invoked to authorise the deployment of the South African National Defence Forces (SANDF) to help fight the spread of COVID-19 (The Constitution, of the Republic of South Africa, 1996a, 1996b; Republic of South Africa, 2002). A significant measure was the imposition of night-time curfews patrolled by the police and the army between 8 pm and 5 am (Heywood, 2020). While the curfews were instituted for public health ends and to save lives, they caused serious tensions with the "fundamental democratic freedoms" (Vasilopoulos et al., 2022:1). Several episodes of lockdowns with adjustments were introduced, supported by the scaling up of personal protective equipment (PPE) distribution and intensive care unit (ICU) bed capacity in hospitals. Section 27 of the SA Constitution regarding the right to social security informed the provision of COVID-19 relief in the form of financial and material support for those whose livelihoods were disrupted by the lockdown measures (Hofman & Madhi, 2020).

While the GoS tried to respond to COVID-19 within the bounds of the constitution and international human rights laws, the military-supported lockdown measures were characterised by the excessive use of force. Another quagmire was that relaxing the approaches to lockdowns was likely to promote the surge of infection figures and in the end, the GoS was going to be labelled negligent. Consequently, lockdown measures had to be enforced with or without citizen consent, a decision described by Herbert and Marquette (2021: 7) as "emergency politics". It is fair to say that the COVID-19 pandemic created not only panic but also a moral dilemma in the governance of health pandemics.

Human rights abuses during the COVID-19 lockdown enforcement in South Africa

The GoS earned its fair share of condemnation regarding human rights violations during the enforcement of lockdown measures. Numerous reports of human rights violations nationwide militated against the proactive measures instituted to combat the pandemic. Amnesty International, a human rights watchdog, reported on the incidence of the South African Police Service (SAPS) and SANDF brutality toward citizens for failing to comply with lockdown regulations. A striking revelation is that between 25 March and 5 May 2020, the Independent Investigative Policy Directorate (IPID) reportedly received an estimated 828 complaints against the policy (Amnesty International Report, 2020). Related documented evidence on police brutality, talks about over 589 cases of rape, and 32 deaths in police custody were reported. (Amnesty International Report, 2020). The most gruesome murder cases are that of Collins Khosa and Nathaniel Jules. The former was allegedly beaten to death by the SANDF on 10 April 2020 in the Alexandra township of Johannesburg for allegedly violating lockdown regulations (Amnesty International Report, 2020). The latter, a 16-year-old disabled boy from Eldorado Park, was reportedly shot by the police at a nearby shop for failure to answer certain questions because he was deaf (Amnesty International Report, 2020; Kanjeni, 2020). Sibusiso Amos from Vosloorus reportedly died at the hands of Ekhuruleni Metro Police for alleged non-compliance with COVID-19 regulations (Pettersson, 2020).

There are well-documented incidents of people being whipped with sjamboks by SAPS in high-density areas like Khayelitsha, Hillbrow, Masiphumelele, Yeoville, and Makanza (Pettersson, 2020). Other appalling reports pertain to the eviction of illegal dwellers in Makanza, Cape Town, using rubber bullets and tear gas (Cilliers, 2021; Friedman, 2020). Reported also are incidents of citizens in informal settlements and slums being forced to frog-jump and kicked on their backs by some SAPS members (Ciliiers, 2021). These violations are described by Bresciani and Hughes (2020: 1) as "virological witch hunts", thus, depicting mindless attacks on the innocent by the state security forces and highlighting the irresponsible protection by the state security agents and a manifest failure of R2P on the part of the GoS.

There is also an element of leadership ethics and responsibility in the commission of COVID-19–instigated human rights violations. This can be argued in the context of the use of inflammatory language and endorsement of tacit measures by Minister of Police Beki Cele and the then Minister of Defence Nosiwe Masipa-Nqakula. The Minister of Police brazenly endorsed the use of force arguing that "we have to push and nudge them towards obeying the law" (SABC News, 2020: 1). Cele went on to describe the police as "being kind" to those found contravening lockdown measures (SABC News, 2020: 1). Similarly, Masipa-Nqakula justified the use of coercive measures by the SANDF to make "people understand fully the dangers of getting the virus" (Farr & Green, 2020).

The heavy-handedness of the lockdown enforcement and the human rights disaster prompted the UN to demand an end to the "toxic lockdown enforcement culture" (UN News, 2020). A human rights deficit in the enforcement of lockdown regulations in the townships and informal settlements attracted condemnation for inflicting serious suffering on the already impoverished. Measures to eliminate "super spreaders" imploded on the poor's livelihoods, especially street vending, job searching on the roads, and seeking better services and amenities (Bueno de Mesquita et al., 2021; Defenceweb, 2020). For a country characterised by acute poverty and inequalities, one would expect the GoS to implement lockdowns in a pro-poor and responsible manner. Thus Hofman and Madh (2020) questioned whether the SAPS and SANDF were serving a legitimate purpose.

The role of SAPS and SANDF in enforcing lockdown measures seemingly disregarded international humanitarian laws and the UN Convention on Civil and Political Rights. Measures instituted to promote public health fall short of proportionality and limitedness. Bueno de Mesquita et al. (2021) exposed the missing link between human rights protection and COVID-19 policing. They claim that while COVID-19 responses required limiting economic, social, and cultural rights, the measures should have been proportionate to the danger being addressed and should be specifically for public health promotion. Ironically, the implementation of the lockdown was arbitrary and discriminatory in orientation because people in the medium-density residential areas did not experience the same (Bueno de Mesquita et al., 2021). Regardless of the public health benefits of the lockdown measures, the fact that the vulnerable and the marginalised of society were most affected waters down the GoS's commitment to R2P. Precisely, the practicality of complying with the lockdown measures in contexts of informal settlements and townships where people share one common communal tap for water attracted condemnation (Buthelezi, 2020). As noted by Levine and Menderson (2020), with no basic income, the poor in these localities who survive on street vending, spaza shops, and menial jobs were bound to breach the lockdown regulations to fend for their families. Again, the food parcels rendered by the GoS and well-wishers were arguably not adequate to sustain livelihoods (Buthelezi, 2020).

The appalling COVID-19 human rights violations culminated in the breakdown of the social contract and public confidence in the state and its security clusters. By violating the rights of the citizens merely for failure to observe lockdown regulations, the government failed to provide adequate justification that the measures were in the interest of the public. In a reproach statement, the former public protector, Professor Thuli Madonsela, questioned the reasonableness of enforcement of lockdown laws. She challenged that "laws must also be just, fair and reasonable in the court of public opinion" (Madonsela, 2020: 2). The message is explicit that public policies and conduct should conform to moral standards and not only in the court of law (Hofman & Madji, 2020). Critics further lament the crude methods of curfews characterised by troop deployment on streets, which resembles a situation of a state at war with its citizens (Cooper & Aitchison, 2020; Herbert & Marquette, 2021).

The criticism marshalled on the GoS pertains to the irrational implementation of the lockdown measures especially, deviating from the precepts of the constitution of the land, the Bill of Rights, and the ethos of *ubuntu* regarding the protection of human rights and freedoms. Advancing the right to protection from the pandemic seemingly overshadowed the rule of law and several facets of human rights to be enjoyed by the citizens. Hofman and Madji (2020), cites section 36 of the Constitution of South Africa, regarding the Bill of Rights to show that lockdown enforcement measures failed to conform with the constitutional provisions regarding the protection of the citizens. The Bill of Rights emphatically states that the limitation of human rights in times of pandemics is "reasonable and justified in an open and democratic society based on human dignity, equality and freedom" (Constitution of the Republic of South Africa Bill of Rights, Section 36: 1996). Similarly, the Siracusa Principles regarding the state of emergency adopted by the 1984 UN Economic and Social Council decrees that "any measures taken to protect the population that limit people's rights and freedoms must be lawful, necessary and proportionate" (Ramcharan, 2011). Reasonably so, the protection of the right to health should not eclipse other rights provided by the global Universal Declaration of Human Rights in 1948.

The decision to invoke criminal law to enforce civilian compliance during lockdown enforcement further exposed the conflictual relationship between human rights protection and lockdown enforcement (Bueno de Mesquita et al., 2021). That explains why any failure to comply with the measures attracted criminalisation of violations, as evidenced by the reports on arbitrary arrests and several human rights abuses. To show that human rights protection in COVID-19 mitigation evaded policymakers, the C-19 People's Coalition, a civic movement against repression by the state security clusters during COVID-19, raised concern over the Parliamentary Portfolio Committee on COVID-119, challenging the suspension of the Bill of Rights. The movement cited incidents of draconian approaches to lockdown by the SAPS, SANDF, and municipal police service (Pettersson, 2020). The unethical and illegal conduct by the arms of the law prompted Sikkink (2020: 1) to remind us that while "protecting our collective right to health", there is a need to "balance our individual rights". Irresponsible protection by the SAPS and SANDF further contradicted the address to the nation on 26 March 2020, by President Cyril Ramaphosa that stated security forces were merely "to support and guide people to comply with the lockdown regulations" Pettersson, (2020: 1). Interestingly, the joint SAPS-SANDF ended up waging war against the citizens and to a larger extent deviated from the mandate of saving lives.

Juxtaposing the human rights realisation and lockdown enforcement balance

Inadvertently, the military-police nexus, in the implementation of lockdown measures, authored the recession in human rights protection and upholding democratic values in the country. The phenomenon of governance through a military style is not new to the country. Evidence shows that the adoption of military methods and the use of force to guide citizen policing has some colonial traits (Lamb, 2018; Burger, 2012). During the apartheid system, joint SAPS-SANDF operations were utilised to crush civil dissent in the townships (Lamb, 2018). Despite the transition from apartheid to democracy in 1994, re-militarisation of the police surfaced in 2010 when the SAPS ranks were reoriented along military lines (Lamb, 2018; Hornberger, 2013; Burger, 2012). Militarisation of the police is evidenced by embracing titles such as "colonel" and "general and brigadier" (Burger, 2012). While the trans-formation was informed by the desire to step up to the escalating crime, waging a war type of response led to the inevitable outcome of the erosion of professionalism and human rights violations. That is because military ideals characterised by using excessive force became a defining mode of operation. The police brutality that culminated in the Marikana killings in 2012 is a test case of the entrenched military conduct of the SAPS (Lamb, 2018). Later, the velocity and intensity of COVID-19 triggered a similar government-sanctioned military response, with serious human rights abuses. The establishment of the NCCC again received criticism for carrying tones of militarisation in COVID-19 responses. Haffajee (2020: 1) laments that the term "command" resonates with a war-like situation and does not conform to the ideals of "democracy, servant leadership and public health promotion". The idea of establishing NCCC, though initially for COVID-19 combative purposes, is criti-cised for advancing the centralisation of power and that made it permissible to vio-late human rights and freedoms. The pressing question posed by Haffajee (2020:1) therefore is "who guards the guardians"? Implicitly, the SANDF and SAPS were al-lowed to implement lockdown measures without any checks and balances, and that positions COVID-19 responses in an uneasy relationship with the international R2P norms and domestic laws regarding human rights protection. It could be argued that while the GoS delivered on its duty to protect people from the COVID-19 virus, subjecting the same to unnecessary torture, killings, and wanton human rights viola-tions becomes an oxymoron.

Based on the preceding discussion, it could be argued that the unethical con-duct by the police and the army during lockdown enforcement proved counterpro-ductive. Measures instituted during COVID-19 enforcement were partial, as they advanced the ends of public health while suffocating the fundamental rights and freedoms of the citizens. A critical apprehension is the erosion of basic human rights reminiscent of the apartheid times. The blended civil-military engagement in SA lacked established "parameters and limits to their involvement" (Gibson-Fall, 2021: 6). That also accounts for the breakdown in the social contract and souring of civil-military relations in the country. Overall, the military involvement had serious hu-man rights repercussions, and that exposes GoS's ordeal with R2P, the Bill of Rights, and other international human rights laws. Notably, the 2005 International Health Regulations obligates states to uphold human rights in their response to global pan-demics. That considers the respect for human dignity, rights, and freedoms (WHO, 2005). In the SA case, these measures were flouted despite the existence of a sound constitution and the president's pledge to uphold the Bill of Rights and human rights during lockdown enforcement.

Quite revealing is that by deploying the SANDF and SAPS, the GoS considered limiting basic rights the appropriate measure to curb the spread of COVID-19. Consequently, the imbalance between lockdown enforcement and upholding hu-man rights exposed the GoS's lack of a human rights–based approach to fighting COVID-19. Evidently, by authorising the SANDF and the SAPS to use coercive measures to force civilian compliance, the GoS seemingly suspended international human rights principles merely because of the pandemic and licensed irresponsible conduct by the state security apparatus. For a country battling to come to terms with memories of the 2012 Marikana killings, where 34 mineworkers were killed by the police, the GoS ought to have outlawed the use of firearms and excessive force for lockdown enforcement. The Human Rights Watch (2020: 2) submits that the UN Charter obliges governments to take measures to "prevent, treat and control the spread of endemic and pandemic diseases". While restrictions on some rights are justifiable based on scientific evidence of how the COVID-19 virus spread, government responses should, however, carefully consider basic human rights and dignity in delivering on the duty to protect. Thus, the complementarity between basic human rights and the right to health should have been harnessed.

Conclusion

The chapter discussed the human rights protection crisis in South Africa during the COVID-19 pandemic. It argues that the pandemic presented the GoS with the challenge of delivering on its R2P mandate as evidenced by fraught lockdown policing measures that infringed on some of the citizens' constitutional rights including the right to life. The chapter revealed that a human rights–based approach to lockdown implementation should have appealed to SA, given that the country endured a long history of human rights suppression propelled by institutionalised racial discrimination. The non-alignment of lockdown measures and human rights protection, therefore, invoked memories of the apartheid era characterised by restrictions on human freedoms. On the other hand, the chapter demonstrated that human rights protection in times of public health crises is a mission impossible. If the SA government had to relax its approach to lockdown implementation at the height of the COVID-19 pandemic, the protection obligation was going to be rendered obsolete since the pandemic is virulent. On the other hand, using tacit measures as evidenced by the militarised lockdown enforcement attracts questions about responsibility while protecting. Fundamentally, curfews and the draconian approach to lockdown measures signify a regression in democracy and human rights consolidation in the country.

The fact that the country is the last colonial outpost in Southern Africa and endured prolonged human rights violations under the apartheid system creates the imperative for balancing human rights and lockdown enforcement measures. The unequivocal question that evaded the policymakers as discussed pertains to who needs to be protected and from what or who. Analysing the handling of the lockdown enforcement through the prism of R2P demonstrated that the imperative for responsible protection in times of pandemics or public health crises is nonnegotiable. Arguably, it is the GoS's national responsibility to protect its citizens from all avoidable harm and at the same time uphold the rule of law and human rights protection laws. The chapter recommends the adoption of human rights–based approaches to respond to future global pandemics and responsible protection to avoid snuffing out people's basic rights and freedoms.

References

Amnesty International Report. 2020. *The State of the World's Human Rights; South Africa 2020.* https://www.ecoi.net/en/document/2048756.html

Bachelet, M. 2020. COVID-19: States should not abuse emergency measures to suppress human rights – UN experts. *UN-Commissioner for Humana Rights: Press Release*, 27 April. www.ohchr.org/en/statements/2020/04/covid-19-exceptional-measures-should-not-be-cover-human-rights-abuses-and

Bekema, J. D. L. C. 2021. Pandemics and the punitive regulation of the weak: Experiences of COVID-19 survivors from urban poor communities in the Philippines. *Third World Quarterly*, 42(8): 1679–1695.

Bresciani, C. and Hughes, G. 2020. *Virological Witch Hunts: Coronavirus and Social Control under Quarantine in Bergamo, Italy.* https://boasblogs.org/witnessingcorona/virological-witch-hunts/

Bueno de Mesquita, J., Kapilashrami, A. and Meier, B. M. 2021. *Human Rights Dimensions of the COVID-19 Pandemic.* Colchester: The Independent Panel for Pandemics Preparedness and Responses, University of Essex. https://repository.essex.ac.uk/31127/1/Background-paper-11-Human-rights.pdf

Burger, J. 2012. To what extent has the South African police service become Militarised? *Institute of Security Studies Today*, 6 December. https://issafrica.org/iss-today/to-what-extent-has-the-south-african-police-service-become-militarised

Buthelezi, M. 2020. *South Africa, COVID-19 and the Social Contract, Public Affairs Research Institute.* https://pari.org.za/south-africa-covid-19-social-contract/

Cilliers, C. 2021. 'Who's fooling who?' ANC roasted for 'breaching' lockdown regulations. *The Citizen*, 27 September. www.citizen.co.za/news/south-africa/elections/local-2021/2633548/whos-fooling-who-anc-roasted-for-breaching-lockdown-regulations/

The Constitution, of the Republic of South Africa. 1996a. *As Adopted on 8 May 1996 and Amended on 11 October 1996 by the Constitutional Assembly.* www.justice.gov.za/legislation/constitution/saconstitution-web-eng.pdf

The Constitution, of the Republic of South Africa. 1996b. *Chapter 2 Bill of Rights.* www.justice.gov.za/legislation/constitution/SAConstitution-web-eng-02.pdf

Constitution of the Republic of South Africa Bill of Rights 1996. Parliament, Cape Town. https://www.gov.za/documents/constitution/chapter-2-bill-rights

Cooper, L. and Aitchison, G. 2020. *The Dangers Ahead: COVID-19, Authoritarianism and Democracy.* London: London School of Economics (LSE) Conflict and Civil Society Research Unit.

Cooper, L. and Aitchison, G. 2021. *The Dangers Ahead: Covid-19, Authoritarianism and Democracy.* London: London School of Economics (LSE) Conflict and Civil Society Research Unit.

Davies, S. E. 2008. Securitizing infectious disease. *International Affairs*, 84(2): 295–313.

De Waal, A. 2010. Reframing governance, security and conflict in the light of HIV/AIDS: A synthesis of findings from the AIDS, security and conflict initiative. *Social Science & Medicine*, 70(1): 114–120.

De Waal, A., Klot, J., Mahajan, M., Huber, D., Frerks, G. and M'Boup, S. 2010. *HIV/AIDS, Security and Conflict: New Realities, New Responses*. The Hague, Netherlands: SSRC/Clingendael Institute for ASCI.

DefenceWeb. 2020. *Draconian Lockdown Measures in SA – UN Human Rights, Commissioner*, 29 April. www.defenceweb.co.za/featured/draconian-lockdown-measures-in-sa-un-human-rights-commissioner/

Elbe, S. 2006. Should HIV/AIDS be securitized? The ethical dilemmas of linking HIV/AIDS and security. *International Studies Quarterly*, 50(1): 119–144.

Evans, G. 2008. The responsibility to protect: An idea whose time has come . . . and gone? *International Relations*, 22(3): 283–298.

Friedman, S. 2020. South Africa's lockdown: A great start, but then a misreading of how society works. *The Conversation*, 4 June. https://theconversation.com/south-africas-lockdown-a-great-start-but-then-a-misreading-of-how-society-works-139789

Gibson-Fall, F. 2021. Military responses to COVID-19, emerging trends in global civil-military engagements. *Review of International Studies*, 47(2): 155–170.

Greer, S. L., King, E. J., da Fonseca, E. M. and Peralta-Santos, A. 2020. The comparative politics of COVID-19: The need to understand government responses. *Global Public Health*, 15(9): 1413–1416.

Guterres, A. 2021. The world faces a pandemic of human rights abuses in the wake of COVID-19. *The Guardian*, p. 22.

Haffajee, F. 2020. National Coronavirus Command Council: Who guards the guardians? *The Daily Maverick*, 7 May. https://www.dailymaverick.co.za/article/2020-05-07-national-coronavirus-command-council-who-guards-the-guardians/

Harman, S. and Wenham, C. 2018. Governing Ebola: Between global health and medical humanitarianism. *Globalizations*, 15(3): 362–376.

Herbert, S. and Marquette, H. 2021. *COVID-19, Governance, and Conflict: Emerging Impacts and Future Evidence Needs. K4D Emerging Issues Report 34*. Brighton: Institute of Development Studies.

Heywood, M. 2020. Human rights, the rule of law, and COVID-19 in South Africa. *Bill of Health*. https://blog.petrieflom.law.harvard.edu/2020/06/04/south-africa-global-responses-covid19

Hofman, K. and Madhi, S. 2020. The unanticipated costs of COVID-19 to South Africa's quadruple disease burden. *South African Medical Journal*, 110(8): 698–699.

Hornberger, J. 2013. From general to commissioner to general – on the popular state of policing in South Africa. *Law and Social Inquiry*, 38(3): 598–614.

Hosken, G. 2021. Amnesty International Slams SA for violating citizens' rights under lockdown. *The Timeslive Online*. https://www.timeslive.co.za/news/south-africa/2021-04-27-amnesty-international-slams-sa-for-violating-citizens-rights-under-lockdown/

Human Rights Watch (HRW). 2020. *Human Rights Dimensions of COVID-19 Responses*. New York. www.hrw.org/news/2020/03/19/human-rights-dimensions-covid-19-response.

International Commission on Intervention and State Sovereignty (ICISS). 2001. *The Responsibility to Protect Report*. Ottawa, Canada: International Development Research.

Jarvis, S. 2020. The responsibility to protect in 2020: Thinking beyond the UN security council. *E-International Relations*. www.e-ir.info/2020/06/19/the-responsibility-to-protect-in-2020-thinking-beyond-the-un-security-council/ (accessed 29 December 2021).

Jeiroudi, N. 2021. The wrath of a pandemic: A call to expand R2P in response to Covid-19. *Michigan Journal of International Law* 42. mjilonline.org

Kanjeni, U. 2020. Justice for nathaniel julies: What you need to know about the teen's dearth. *The Times*, 28 August. www.timeslive.co.za/news/south-africa/2020-08-28-justice-for-nathaniel-julius-what-you-need-to-know-about-the-teens-death/

Lamb, G. 2018. Police militarisation and the 'war on crime' in South Africa. *Journal of Southern African Studies*, 44(5): 933–949.

Levine, S. and Manderson, L. 2020. The militarisation of the COVID-19 response in South Africa (#WitnessingCorona). *Medizinethnologie.net*, 9 April. www.medizinethnologie.net/the-militarisation-of-the-covid-19-response-in-south-africa/

Li, Y. and Galea, S. 2020. Racism and the COVID-19 epidemic: Recommendations for health care workers. *American Journal of Public Health*, 110(7): 956.

Madonsela, T. 2020. Thuli Madonsela: An open letter to Cyril Ramaphosa. *Financial Mail*, 4 June. https://www.businesslive.co.za/fm/opinion/protected-space/2020-06-04-thuli-madonsela-an-open-letter-to-cyril-ramaphosa/

Mawarire, T. 2020. Things will never be the same again. COVID-19 effects on freedom of expression in Southern Africa. *2020 Research Report. Internews: Local Voices-Global Change.*

National Institute of Communicable Diseases. 2020. *First Case of COVID-19 Coronavirus Reported in SA*, 5 March. www.nicd.ac.za/first-case-of-covid-19-coronavirus-reported-in-sa/

Peak, T. 2020. *Is There a Responsibility to Protect the World from Pandemics?* Centre for Geopolitics, University of Cambridge.

Pettersson, T. J. 2020. *Submission to Portfolio Committee on Police Concerning the Use of Force by the SAPS in the Implementation of Regulations Made in Terms of the Disaster Management Act, People's Coalition.* https://static.pmg.org.za/200429C19_submission.pdf

Ramcharan, B. G. 2011. The Siracusa Principles. In *The Fundamentals of International Human Rights Treaty Law*, pp. 223–238. Leiden: Brill Nijhoff.

Republic of South Africa. 1996. *Constitution of the Republic of South Africa*. Cape Town: Parliament of the Republic of South Africa.

Republic of South Africa. 2002. *Defence Act-Act 42*. Government *Gazette*. Cape Town: Parliament of the Republic of South Africa.

Sikkink, K. 2020. Rights and responsibilities in the Coronavirus pandemic. *OpenGlobalRights. org.* www.openglobalrights.org/rights-and-responsibilities-in-the-coronavirus-pandemic/

Smith, K. 2020. A reflection on the responsibility to protect in 2020. *Global Centre for the Responsibility to Protect.* https://reliefweb.int/sites/reliefweb.int/files/resources/2020-July-Smith.pdf (accessed 29 December 2021).

South African Broadcast Cooperation News (SABC News). 2020. National Command Council give update on COVID-19 lockdown. *SABC News*, 27 March. https://www.youtube.com/watch?v=YLRCsndfpHg

South African Government News Agency (SA News). 2021. *Over 2 000 SANDF Members Deployed to Help Fight COVID-19*, January 20. www.sanews. gov.za/south-africa/over-2-000-sandf-members-deployed-help-fight-covid-19

South African Government Press Release. 2022. Minister Joe Phaahla: Repeal of regulations regarding COVID-19 pandemic and monkey-pox, 23 June 2022. www.gov.za/speeches/statement-minister-health-dr-joe-phaahla-repeal-regulations-notifiable-medical-conditions

Thakur, R. 2016. The responsibility to protect at 15. *International Affairs*, 92(2): 415–434.

United Nations. 2005. *World Summit Outcome – Resolution Adopted by the General Assembly A/RES/60/1* (resolution 60/1, 2005). https://undocs.org/A/RES/60/1

United Nations Development Programme (UNDP). 1994. *Human Development Report 1994: New Dimensions of Human Security*. New York: United Nations Development Programme.

United Nations Economic and Social Council. 1984. *The Siracusa Principles, Commission on Human Rights, Decision 104, Status of the International Covenants on Human Rights*. Geneva: United Nations Economic and Social Council.

United Nations News (UN News). 2020. *News in Brief*, 27 April. https://news.un.org/en/audio/2020/04/1062652

United Nations Office of the High Commissioner on Human Rights (UNOHCHR). 2020. *COVID-19: States Should Not Abuse Emergency Measures to Suppress Human Rights–UN Experts*. Geneva.

United Nations Sustainable Development Goals. 2015. *Transforming our World: The 2030 Agenda for Sustainable Development*. New York, NY: United Nations.

Vasilopoulos, P., McAvay, H., Brouard, S. and Foucault, M. 2022. The fregility of democratic freedoms in the COVID-19 pandemic. *The Loop*. https://theloop.ecpr.eu/the-fragility-of-civil-liberties-during-the-covid-19-pandemic/

Wambua, M. 2020. COVID-19, Human Security and the Responsibility to Protect. *Social Science Research Council*, Brooklyn NY, USA. https://kujenga-amani.ssrc.org/2020/09/03/covid-19-human-security-crisis-and-the-responsibility-to-protect/

Watterson, C. and Kamradt-Scott, A. 2016. Fighting flu: Securitization and the military role in combating influenza. *Armed Forces & Society*, 42(1): 145–168.

Wenham, C. and Farias, D. B. 2019. Securitizing Zika: The case of Brazil. *Security Dialogue*, 50(5): 398–415.

Williams, C. R., Kestenbaum, J. G. and Meier, B. M. 2020. Populist nationalism threatens health and human rights in the COVID-19 response. *American Journal of Public Health*, 110(12): 1766–1768.

World Health Organization (WHO). 2005. *International Health Regulations* – No. SEA/RC58/R4. Geneva, Switzerland: World Health Organization. https://apps.who.int/iris/bitstream/handle/10665/204408/rc58_r4.pdf

World Health Organization (WHO). 2020. *WHO Director-General's Opening Remarks at the Media Briefing on COVID-19 – 11 March 2020*. Geneva, Switzerland. WHO Director-General's opening remarks at the media briefing on COVID-19 – 22 December 2021.

World Health Organization (WHO). 2022. *WHO Coronavirus (COVID-19) Dashboard*, 5 July. https://covid19.who.int/region/afro/country/za

Zwane, T. 2020. 76% of South Africa's businesses report revenue loss as COVID-19 bites. *City Press*, 20 September. www.news24.com/citypress/business/76-of-south-africas-businesses-report-revenue-loss-as-covid-19-bites-20200902

7

A TROJAN HORSE

Critically exploring data as a colonial instrument during the COVID-19 pandemic in South Africa

Kyle John Bester and Danille Elize Arendse

Introduction

The Trojan horse was created by the Greeks to surreptitiously convey their soldiers into Troy, as they had been struggling to gain entry into the fortified city. The Trojans believed that the wooden horse was a gift and opened their gates to let it in. This deception, through the wooden horse strategy used by the Greeks, became known as a Trojan horse (Encyclopaedia Britannica, 2018). An anti-apartheid protest was staged by students on 15 October 1985 in Athlone.[1] On this day, the police arranged with the railway officials to hide in a railway carriage that had crates on it, so that they would not be visible. The railway carriage then drove through the protesters and, once in sight of the protesters, the police exposed themselves and shot at the youth using live ammunition. During this incident, three youths were killed and several injured. This incident became known as the Trojan Horse Massacre (South African History Online, 2020). Many years later, another Trojan horse appeared, but in the form of a computer virus. These Trojan horses (computer codes) are often added to a computer without the user's knowledge when they are either downloading free software or while perusing the internet. This Trojan horse observes the user's online activities and transmits the information to the hacker who created the Trojan horse, who now has access to the user's information and may control any information on the user's computer remotely (Pandya, 2013).

The authors used the analogy of the Trojan horse as the theme of this chapter. Data, the new Trojan horse, wraps itself in the desires of the human being and presents itself as a reward to fill their lives with joy. In this way, people become enslaved in a new system, which the authors of this chapter and others call data colonialism (Couldry & Mejias, 2019a). Data colonialism can be defined as "an emerging order for the appropriation of human life so that data can be continuously extracted from it for profit"

DOI: 10.4324/9781003415121-7

(Couldry & Mejias, 2019a: *xiii*). This facilitates the notion that data is a contemporary commodity in capitalism (Couldry & Mejias, 2019b; Van der Spuy, 2020). This emerging order has long-term consequences that may be as far-reaching as the historical appropriations carried out by colonialism for the benefit of the capitalist economies and the legislative order that subsequently developed internationally.

In this chapter the authors present the argument that data colonialism is a new form of colonialism operating in the world today. Therefore, when considering the history of colonialism and apartheid in South Africa (Piotrowski, 2019; Mariotti & Fourie, 2014; Ogura, 1996; Terreblanche, 1994), it is necessary to integrate this history with the way that data colonialism may be emerging in this country as a new form of colonialism (Couldry & Mejias, 2019a, b). In this context, data is viewed as a resource and a tool for advancing capitalism (Couldry & Mejias, 2019b). It is evident, through a data colonialism lens (Couldry & Mejias, 2019b), how data is continuing the goals of historical colonialism and apartheid in South Africa. Although the violence associated with colonialism and apartheid is not the same, violence is nevertheless present in data colonialism (Couldry & Mejias, 2019a, b). Having said this, this chapter argues that during the COVID-19 pandemic, data colonialism was accelerated. However bleak this reality may appear, it presents the opportunity to decolonise and re-create our reality. This chapter therefore argues for the advancement of social justice in South Africa, where data colonialism is threatening the freedom and equality of the people.

Colonialism and apartheid in South Africa

There's a land grab occurring right now, and it's for your data and your freedom: companies are not only surveilling you, they're increasingly influencing and controlling your behaviour . . . the new colonialism at the heart of modern computing and serves as a needed wake up call to everyone who cares about our future relationship with technology.

(Schneier, 2015 in Couldry & Mejias, 2019a)

The aforementioned quote aptly refers to colonialism and relates specifically to the dispossession of land owned by indigenous South Africans during colonialism and apartheid (Piotrowski, 2019; Mariotti & Fourie, 2014; Ogura, 1996; Terreblanche, 1994). Although the colonial and apartheid empires have ended, the remnants of these empires are still evident in society. These remnants can be argued to have assumed a different form, a technological one, in the data empire era. For this reason, a brief look into South African colonial and apartheid history is crucial for contextualising data colonialism in South Africa.

The four colonisations of South Africa

The past South Africa presents us with an opportunity to revisit how colonialism shaped and continues to shape modern South Africa. In South Africa, there are four consecutive phases in which the country was colonised. The first was labelled an "unofficial colonisation" because African people from different parts of Africa migrated towards South Africa (Piotrowski, 2019; Oliver & Oliver, 2017). This migration was accompanied by the displacement and annihilation of indigenous people as migrants claimed land and settled permanently (Piotrowski, 2019; Oliver & Oliver, 2017). The second colonial movement, however, included the colonisation of both the indigenous people and the African migrants and settlers. This colonial period included Roman-Dutch law, the Reformed religion, capitalism, and slavery (including the concept of servants), which were all absorbed in the way that the Dutch ruled the Cape Colony. Britain, however, conquered the colony from the Dutch in 1806 and officially made it a British colony. This was the third colonisation that South Africa experienced, which lasted until 1961 (Piotrowski, 2019; Oliver & Oliver, 2017; Terreblanche, 1994). The colonial government ensured that the Black labourers were inexpensive and dependent on the money they earned, and the colonial government expropriated large portions of land from the Africans (Piotrowski, 2019; Mariotti & Fourie, 2014; Ogura, 1996; Terreblanche, 1994). Milner's reconstruction policy created a major basis on which land and Black labour succumbed to white capitalism for the economic benefit of only the latter. More importantly, it ensured white dominance over Black people. In this way, a system of racial capitalism and segregation was created. White people (both the English and Afrikaners) benefitted economically from the legally enforced racial capitalism (Piotrowski, 2019; Mariotti & Fourie, 2014; Ogura, 1996; Terreblanche, 1994). The official apartheid governance started in 1948 and only ended in 1994. This colonisation, the fourth colonisation in South Africa, was referred to as "internal colonisation" (Piotrowski, 2019; Oliver & Oliver, 2017). Through Dutch, British, and Afrikaner rule, white supremacy, segregation, racism, separate development, and domination were furthered for economic reasons (Piotrowski, 2019; Isaacs-Martin, 2018; Mariotti & Fourie, 2014; Ogura, 1996; Terreblanche, 1994).

The plagues during colonial South Africa and the COVID-19 pandemic in South Africa

An outbreak of bubonic plague in the year 1901 led to the forced removal of Black (excluding those classified as Coloured and Indian) people from District Six and the docklands area in Cape Town (Sambumbu, 2010). This outbreak of the plague gave the police and government officials an excuse for being armed when they entered District Six (Sambumbu, 2010). The Black people referred to here were relocated to an area called Ndabeni (Kwa-Ndabeni) and were constantly involuntary monitored, their movements and behaviour studied and captured using notebooks and cameras (Sambumbu, 2010). Similarly, in 1904, there was a pneumonic plague outbreak in Johannesburg, South Africa (Evans et al., 2018). It was believed that the plague may have entered South Africa through the rice imported from Bombay, India, at that junction of history. The measures put in place during this period were isolation for infected persons, and the Indian area (identified as having the highest concentration of the disease) was inspected for additional cases and movement was restricted through the use of passes (Evans et al., 2018). Adding to the negative situation, the Indian area was burnt down (as part of actions to alleviate the fears of the white people), and all Black people (inclusive of all classifications) were forced to relocate to an area outside of Johannesburg, the South Western Townships, today better known as Soweto (Evans et al., 2018).

In post-apartheid South Africa, the divide-and-rule strategy continues to advance divisive politics and further the socio-economic divide across race groups (Isaacs-Martin, 2018). When considering how colonialism and apartheid controlled the freedom of movement of Black people, the authors must caution against how COVID-19 may introduce similar control not only over the Black person's body but also over the body of the person who is ill. In this manner, legislation such as the Disaster Management Act 57 of 2002 of South Africa allows for the restriction of movement and use of law enforcement agencies to control the movement of people within South Africa. Furthermore, the COVID-19 pandemic introduced curfews and police brutality similar to what was practised in respect of Black people during apartheid and at the time of the pneumonic plague in Cape Town and Johannesburg, South Africa (Stuurman, 2020; Evans et al., 2018). For this reason, the COVID-19 pandemic in South Africa should be viewed through multiple lenses, one of which is data colonialism.

Data colonialism

Colonialism often highlights the notion of exploitation of time and involuntary labour. Data and colonialism have some parallel features such as the exploitation of resources. However, it might be said that data and colonialism are somewhat different in composition. Traditional forms of colonialism thrive in the form of the physical acquisition of resources by conquering the indigenous people and extracting the resources of a country for the economic prosperity of the coloniser, thus promoting inequality (Couldry & Mejias, 2019a). Data colonialism advances the notion of human exploitation and subliminally encourages a divide through the so-called means of connectivity. As a result, the human is but an element in a constant cycle of "tracking," an entanglement with the facets of space and time. Capitalism focuses on commodities in a social world by directing its attention to human labour. On the other hand, data capitalism focuses on a systemic exchange of power in which users' data is distributed in the form of power in the information-driven world (West, 2019). Couldry and Mejias (2019a) argue that when it comes to the poor and the vulnerable, digital "inclusion" comes at the cost of extensive data profiling, including practices that are predatory, discriminatory, exploitative, or simply degrading.

When considering the subtle forms of colonisation in the earlier colonial history of South Africa, the introduction of data to our ordinary lives has, in many ways, come in subtle forms. Although people have been able to communicate perfectly well without technology and data, their reliance on technology to communicate has subtly become an integral part of present-day life. Similarly, our communication through technology and data has changed significantly and influences how we humans communicate and with whom we communicate. People were therefore not formally colonised by data and technology, but instead migrated towards the forms of data and technology that offered us better and easier ways of communicating, obviating distance and location. For those born in the technological age it may someday be difficult to consider that communication without the use of technology and data ever existed. It might be falsely assumed at some stage in the future that technology and data had always enabled communication.

Data colonialism during the COVID-19 pandemic in South Africa

The current COVID-19 pandemic in South Africa presents a pertinent opportunity to question whether the increased use of virtual spaces might allow data to construct a new form of colonialism. New forms of colonialism such as social media platforms exist in modern society are a latter-day fact of life. These technological platforms depend heavily on information and human interaction. Therefore, the amount of time an individual spends on social media and consumes and exchanges information, and thus driving the creation of and urge for colonialism, links with the notion of large-scale appropriation of resources (Couldry & Mejias, 2019a, b). The main assets the colonial powers set out to acquire were large tracts of territory, including their resources and the humans functioning there. The main aim of appropriation in the modern age is acquiring the life of the human being. All the factors constituting an individual, including their behavioural, psychological, and biological well-being, are extracted by means of data. The cycle of data acquisition, involuntarily obtaining it from people, is an emerging form of colonialism and drives the pursuit of new capitalist means to start a different kind of industrial revolution (Couldry & Mejias, 2019a). Exploring the relationship between colonialism and data offers many advantages, as does studying historical forms of colonialism, as they offer great insight into the appropriation of resources and territory as well as the exploitation of humans' bodies (Couldry & Mejias, 2019a).

Certain events in modern history have forced a rethink of the way data is utilised and extracted through social media platforms and search engines such as Google (Kumar et al., 2016). Indeed, it may be assumed that development in this modern age is characterised by a growing technology base in which knowledge and information represent power. Modern forms of colonialism include the scandal of Cambridge Analytica (data mining company) who was involved in exposing 87 million Facebook user accounts without consent and using the data for political campaigning (Lapaire, 2018; Couldry & Mejias, 2019a; González et al., 2019). To make matters worse, this American company also engaged in a colonial-style move by expanding its activities in Africa (Solomon, 2018). Data mining companies provide governments with rich and in-depth information concerning the "middle", those who have neither strong nor weak political beliefs (Solomon, 2018). Psychological and behavioural profiles can be constructed to persuade not just those who have moderate political beliefs but also the lawmakers and politicians, who are in a position to draft and enforce legislation (Solomon, 2018). It is evident that there is an intersection between knowledge and power. Acquiring both knowledge and power in a neo-colonialist drive towards information dominance may prove to be beneficial for the colonial power on the African continent. By utilising the growing technological communication base in Africa, data mining companies such as Cambridge Analytica are able to create psychological profiles that can reveal the behaviour of people. Thus, the use of data and its transnational nature question the traditional parameters of appropriation and necessitate exploring how data may be able to influence thought patterns. The difference between data colonialism and historical colonialism is that appropriation is at the heart of the latter colonialist process. Historical colonialism involves the appropriation of land and the exploitation of human bodies. Nowadays data mining companies are able to exploit the perceptions and opinions of individuals by crafting messages, images, and information on everyday social media platforms such as Facebook and WhatsApp to influence behaviour and decision-making (González et al., 2019; Solomon, 2018). Data is essentially a neo-colonial tool that fuels capitalism and has the ability to comprehensively construct the individual's everyday functioning (Couldry & Mejias, 2019a). Moreover, data demands to be studied from a colonial perspective in the sense that it contains features of mass inequality.

The previous section set the scene for the way that colonialism links with data. In linking the aforementioned two aspects, it should be highlighted that data falls in the category of "'a means to an end". Making this statement, it is important to acknowledge that data is only as valuable as its purpose. Therefore, data is nothing on its own. It is the purpose for which data will be used that needs investigating and the means and the end relating to this information that require critical thought. The exploration of colonialism and data shapes the setting of the sections to follow in this chapter. First, the subsequent section will address the link between data and COVID-19. Thereafter, this link will be used to gauge the impact on South Africa of the datafication concept in a national lockdown or a COVID-induced lockdown.

The link between data and COVID-19

It is perhaps vital at this stage to emphasise that nation-states such as the United States and the UK have engaged in active deployment of surveillance measures in order to maintain national security (Lyon, 2014). Facial recognition by closed-circuit television (CCTV) cameras is one of the sources collecting facial image data, as is the active monitoring of social media accounts (Shan et al., 2007). This monitoring is largely connected with the deterrence of terrorism. Monitoring people's movements and profiles allows security agencies to construct a comprehensive picture of an individual's network (Shan et al., 2007). Rossi (2018) argues that the right to privacy is challenged by the security and interest of nation-states. The narrative linked to security and the protection of people and national interests is enabled by the use of statistical data. Data, in this debate, is but a pawn to make securitised moves in the social sphere. Threats to society are considered to be damning and may pose a challenge to upholding peace and security (Buzan, 1991).

Making the link to the COVID-19 pandemic, the rise in the infection rate sparked South Africa to create and impose security measures of control to curb the spread of the virus (Pillay & Barnes, 2020; Trippe, 2020). COVID-19 has a high infection rate, and the narrative linked to the strategic responses by the legislative domain, including the health domain, relied on data from various South African health entities (Marivate & Combrink, 2020). It must be emphasised that data and the language linked to control measures was instrumental in informing both security and government departments in South Africa (Marivate & Combrink, 2020; Vreÿ & Solomon, 2020).

COVID-19 is regarded as a potential existential threat that has the possibility of disturbing society's natural order. COVID-19 takes the form of a non-traditional threat which requires mobilisation of exceptional measures, which involved the South African National Defence Force (Vreÿ & Solomon, 2020). With COVID-19, data is presented on a daily basis to inform civilians about the potential dangers of the virus (COVID-19 online resource and news portal 2020). While the infection rate has undergone a significant increase in the latter part of 2020, data has been presented on such a basis that it demanded a prolonged lockdown and the restriction of rights under the Disaster Management Act 57 of 2002 (COVID-19 online resource and news portal 2020; South African Government Gazette, 2002).

During September 2020, the president of South Africa referred to a contact-tracing application that was to be launched in order to curb the spread of the COVID-19 virus by informing South African citizens about areas where there is a potentially high rate of infection (COVID-19 online resource and news portal 2020). The president assured the nation that their data would be kept secure throughout the existence of the application and that they should not fear being identified (COVID-19 online resource and news portal 2020). Whereas this may seem to be a giant leap towards embracing technology within the social realm, it poses significant challenges, as it has been shown that governance and regulation of these contact-tracing applications are yet to be demonstrated and may possibly present a threat to the servers collecting users' data (Sun et al., 2020). Contact-tracing applications have some positives attached to it in that they may sustain an individual's sense of safety and security. Furthermore, the use of such applications can drastically decrease the social stigma attached to having COVID-19, as only a general picture is provided to the users, informing them of the "hot spots" to avoid (COVID-19 online resource and news portal 2020). This consequently limits the element of identifying people. Moreover, because of social stigmatisation that is minimised, it is relevant to note that the civil rights of the individual are not infringed due to the tracing application not seeking personal credentials, which would have enabled further scrutiny (Chowdhury et al.,

2019). However, there are cybersecurity risks attached to contact-tracing applications, as they may expose a user's identity in the event of a threat (Sun et al., 2020).

Data and COVID-19 in South Africa

In reference to data colonialism, the tendency exists to determine how historical colonialism is comparable with a contemporary form of colonialism (Couldry & Mejias, 2019a). Instead, data colonialism is regarded as being a contemporary version of exploitation of labour and time. According to Couldry and Mejias (2019a), in contrast to the traditional form of colonialism, which focused on using human labour to advance its imperial dynasties, data colonialism is the display of power using artificial intelligence (AI) and surveillance mechanisms, which are employed as a means of ensuring safety to the securitising agent. Labour and time are important aspects to focus on in considering historical colonialism. South Africa has its roots firmly in a colonialist past, when certain ethnic groups were exploited. The slave trade flourished by exploiting human lives for economic gain (Couldry & Mejias, 2019b). When referring to data colonialism at the same time as historical colonialism, cognisance should be taken of the size and magnitude in which cyberspace facilitates dispossession.

Since the World Health Organization (WHO) has declared the coronavirus to be a pandemic, various African states as well as their counterparts in the West have opted for stricter control measures to mitigate the spread of infection and to flatten the curve (Staunton et al., 2020; Song et al., 2020). Measures such as regulated quarantine and strict lockdown levels were applied across South Africa, therefore limiting physical interaction, and a more active digital presence was recommended for performing daily activities (Savić, 2020). Owing to the limited availability of the coronavirus vaccine, one of the only mechanisms left to people to prevent their falling ill was to engage in altering their personal behaviour and changing the manner in which interaction and communication were carried out (Pillay & Barnes, 2020). Monitoring and seeking information and data about COVID-19 were aspects that people pursued in order to evaluate their health and potential safety. However, the existence of data regarding the virus also meant that people could be informed about the prevailing state of affairs, including the rate of infection in South Africa (Pillay & Barnes, 2020).

The COVID-19 virus has caused mayhem in South African society, with the concept of coronisation sparking the debate on whether Africans can trust European travellers not to spread the coronavirus. It was widely believed that white European travellers had brought the virus to the African continent and that this was just another means of colonisation. The concept of coronisation was created on the basis of the impact it had on the economy and the social sphere of societies (Johnson, 2020). Locally the impact of COVID-19 has changed the manner in which individuals socialise and perform their everyday tasks (Pillay & Barnes, 2020). The demand for new information regarding cyberspace quickly escalated as cyberspace became an

essential tool for functioning during the pandemic, when human movement was se-
verely restricted owing to the lack of treatment for COVID-19 at the initial *outbreak*
(Pillay & Barnes, 2020).

In the book authored in 2020 by Professor Jakkie Cilliers, Africa First, emphasis
is placed on the growing trend of cyber and internet activities on the African continent (Cilliers, 2020). The concept of "leapfrogging" in the book denotes the rapid
advancement of technology introduced on the African continent (Cilliers, 2020).
This is partly due to globalisation and a demand for cost-effective technology and
broadband services (Cilliers, 2020). Social media platforms and search engines were
heavily depended on during the national lockdown in South Africa (Seacom, 2020),
and still are. Labour in the technological age has also shifted to being more digitally
based. This development is in line with the view that new jobs are constructed in
data colonialism and therefore pose a greater threat to equality and to those who are
able to access the internet (Couldry & Mejias, 2019b). South Africa's economic divide is increasing, and there is a growing call for advancing the distribution of wealth
between the wealthy and the poor (Meiring et al., 2018).

Data and racial capitalism

Facial recognition technology has been at the forefront of collecting the personal data
of civilians in states where surveillance programmes are used as a form of securitisation. Racial profiling[2] is a consequence of surveillance programmes sanctioned by
the state. Data colonialism[3] is a neo-capitalist form of appropriating resources (Couldry & Mejias, 2019b; Mezzadra & Neilson, 2017). This means of appropriation is
advancing at a rapid pace as more users are connecting to the internet. Moreover,
the increase in internet and cyberspace usage has been facilitating the growth in data
colonialism and neo-capitalism in the global and local contexts (Cavelty & Wegner,
2020; West, 2019; Couldry & Mejias, 2019b). This section of the chapter argues that
racial capitalism and racial profiling both exist because of data colonialism.

The nature of cyberspace is that it cannot be contained in a natural geographical
context (Cavelty & Wegner, 2020). Instead, this digital space provides a transnational approach in facilitating the sharing of information and permits individuals to
carry out their daily activities despite geographic restrictions. Cyberspace comprises
widespread use of internet-enabled digital devices that operate through networks
(Cilliers, 2020). Data is an important source for surveillance programmes to be effective in states where security organisations such as the police, military, and health
organisations, which maintain peace and safety, are positioned to use profiling technologies in order to safeguard both communities and external borders (Lyon, 2014;
Soucie, 2012).

In addition, Davenport et al. (2011) believe that active policing has largely been
associated with political and economic contexts. Owing to this biased view, law enforcement agencies are more likely to take action when darker-skinned people are
protesting. Data and technology inherently do not discriminate among or against

people. Instead, they promote communication and foster a sense of community (Couldry & Mejia, 2019b). Yet, recent history indicated that predictive policing tools are able to assist law enforcement agencies in targeting and imposing surveillance techniques to identify civilians, based on the traits of their community, as "dangerous" (Koen, 2017). Couldry and Mejias (2019a) argue that colonialism in its rawest form prefers to exploit new territory and requires human bodies to expand economic empires. Data is positioned as a new weapon of power as more individuals are using cyberspace and sharing information on this ephemeral platform. Cyberspace is largely unregulated, which may result in the exploitation of new bodies (personal information). However, it must be stressed that data on its own is not the challenge, but rather the actor that interprets it and uses it, who may exploit those who have innocently shared their personal information in a digital space (Couldry & Mejias, 2019a, b). The trade of human bodies previously took place to advance the economic dominance of colonial powers (Angeles, 2013). The nature of cyberspace and the data attached to it resemble a borderless and transnational state. Therefore, data colonialism in this regard is advanced by the transition to the "new normal," where digital connection is encouraged (Couldry & Mejias, 2019b). The time people allocate to their online activities and the information they seek to retrieve are all used to build a profile of their behaviour and their ways of functioning (Couldry & Mejias, 2019a). From a global perspective, data capitalism has its roots in an e-commerce sector, where online shopping and transactions mainly occur (West, 2017). Data being intrinsic to neo-capitalism is in itself reminiscent of how human labour was utilised in the past to promote the slave trade. The emphasis on capitalism is to conquer new territory where new and unknown resources and bodies could be extracted for labour (Couldry & Mejias, 2019b).

Racial capitalism, however, takes a new turn in the digital era. The personal time that an individual spends in cyberspace and the physical space that is occupied in engaging in a digital sphere are facets of labour in neo-capitalism. These two features, time and space, are a prerequisite when engaging with the so-called new normal (Couldry & Mejias, 2019a). The new normal and the narrative attached to this term has increasingly been highlighted during the COVID-19 period as human labour no longer needs to possess the traits relating to physicality. Instead, physical work and traditional face-to-face contact are aspects that have been discouraged during the so-called new normal. Therefore, from a traditional viewpoint of labour, a core element in the capitalist drive towards monetary advancement now seems to have reached the point when an industrial revolution of a digital nature is imminent. The very nature of cyberspace and the data associated with it have altered the manner in which labour is perceived and performed.

Lever (2016) asserts that racial profiling consists of two reflections, one being a form of statistical discrimination, where generalised characteristics are linked to individuals who are members of a single ethnic group. The second reflection of racial profiling is focused on the notion that societal and racial hierarchy is advanced according to the ethnic features of population groups (Lever, 2016). Facial recognition software and hardware use body cameras, which in the case of protests focus primarily on the collection of facial images of the protesters (Blount, 2017). Facial recognition measures are prone to limitations such as false positives, resulting in the misidentification of Asians and African Americans, which denotes that they might encounter challenges with law enforcement (Access Partnership, 2020). This in itself is a perpetuation of racial inequality and bias through technology. The events of the Black Lives Matter (BLM) protests are a case in point, especially where certain protesters were advocating legal action against law enforcement officials who engaged in brutality (Access Partnership, 2020). The major issue that protesters of colour experienced was that the police were able to identify them and had an extensive profile that extended beyond the normal practical application of law enforcement (Access Partnership, 2020). In many senses, data is a tool that can be viewed as a means to create certainty in uncertain situations (Meijer & Wessels, 2019). Predictive policing and algorithms are used to curb "bad-human" behaviour among population groups that are geographically positioned (Couldry & Mejias, 2019a; Gandy, 2019). Science and technology are utilised in this case to substantiate uncertainty and to calm fears. This creates the impression that militarisation in maintaining and securing peace is necessary and that technology and science have neutral bases. Technology used by the police is in no way created to be neutral. Instead, it depends on the early detection of and issue of alerts about crime and illicit activities in hot spots.

Surveillance mechanisms that use facial recognition technology in collecting data are able to cause problems relating to individual civil rights and privacy (Access Partnership, 2020). If these biometric technologies go unregulated, challenges other than legislation, such as discrimination, may occur (Gandy, 2019). This is owing to the hierarchical nature of racial inequality and injustice, which are sustained through targeting general traits and behaviour (Gandy, 2019). Moreover, when biometric data is not discarded immediately, it may result in rapid cross-referencing of personal information when accessing platforms that require the disclosure of data. The cross-referencing of data (for example, verifying of identification number) may also give way to predict patterns of characteristics and behaviours of individuals living in a specific geographical location (Couldry & Mejias, 2019). The implications of geographical targeting within the predictive analysis of potential threats are certainly racial. Geographical location often becomes an alternative for race and ethnicity (Carter, 2009; Cook & Kemeny, 2017). Machines and its algorithms are able to connect traits with race groups. This concurs in the current era, when predictive policing and science are utilised as justifiable tools to safeguard society against impending threats. In the South African context, this could resemble protecting people against elements of crime and increased violence. Crime and violence are key factors that confirm the legitimacy of accessing, understanding, and monitoring human behaviour (Couldry & Mejias, 2019; Van Dijk, 2014). The danger of quantifying violence and linking it to ethnicity is that crime becomes racialised. The scientific viewpoint, supported by data, permits this data phenomenon (Wang, 2018). In this regard, data creates social and racial segregation and exacerbates narratives of anti-Black and

Black criminality. For South Africans, this is reminiscent of colonialism and apartheid surveillance.

From Buzan's (1991) securitisation point of view, it can be highlighted that the securitising actor is able to recommend emergency measures to the public in order to safeguard peace and maintain normality in society. During 1901, the use of guns and batons were considered necessary tools for maintaining order and to curb the spread of the plague (Sambumbu, 2010). Police brutality against Black people in South Africa is deeply rooted in the legacy of apartheid (Staunton et al., 2020). Much attention was focused on police presence in Black communities in South Africa, which substantiates the idea that crime is still geographically determined (Trippe, 2020). During the course of the national lockdown, at Level 5, it was punishable by law for a person to be seen outside their home (Staunton et al., 2020). Movement was only allowed if there was credible evidence of a person being an essential worker. The same rules applied during apartheid and in the forced removal of people in South Africa, where the freedom of movement of certain people was restricted (Staunton et al., 2020; Trotter, 2019). At the same time, it should be stressed that, in the guise of the National Disaster Act (South African Government Gazette, 2002), the South African National Defence Force (SANDF) was also provided with increased powers to enforce the lockdown laws (Staunton et al., 2020). The militarised response in the country is characteristic of the measures imposed during apartheid-era policing, when movement was restricted and people were relocated against their will (Staunton et al., 2020).

Certain areas and neighbourhoods are associated with the perception that they are unsafe. The technology therefore enables the notion that certain characteristics are associated with a certain race and area. In addition to this, it should be noted that in this crime is racialised (Wang, 2018). However, as can be said with all computerised systems, it depends massively on the human element. The human teaches and trains machines to perform certain tasks. The same applies to algorithms, as humans also create these. Thus, technology and systems that are created are associated with one or another vulnerability. This therefore enhances the perspective that humans are the weak link in the technology chain (Cavelty & Wegner, 2020). The vulnerability in this regard may point to the necessity to teach machines to discriminate between race groups and to discern behavioural traits in population groups (Wang, 2018). Thus, people socially construct crime, and the scientific measures that exist to deal with it are, in some part human, and therefore open to prejudice. A narrative concerning a sense of insecurity needs to be constructed in order for surveillance mechanisms to be implemented. Data, as has been highlighted, is used as a Trojan horse, a shell that masks the intention to create perceived stability and safety (Wang, 2018). The construction of threats ties in with the dynamic of implementing measures that are effective for sustaining security. Therefore, a suitable narrative needs to be constructed by securitising actors (state, state-affiliated actors, and security forces) to recipients (civil society) (Buzan, 1991). The narrative concerning an existential threat must be created and successfully received in civil society so that the threat can be publicly acknowledged (Buzan, 1991). Having said this, COVID-19 in South Africa is constructed as a both a medical emergency and security threat and thus leaves us vulnerable to racial profiling and heightened levels of surveillance and control through the strategic use of our data. As a result, data colonialism makes us susceptible to racial capitalism, as COVID-19 threatens to reproduce social and economic inequalities.

Decolonising data in a South African context

Throughout this chapter arguments have been presented that promote the recognition of data and the digital space as a potential area vulnerable to exploitation and dispassion. In exploring data, there is a need to recognise its colonial and capitalist nature, which may serve to disempower humans and enslave them through different forms of oppression. It is therefore fitting to explore the possibilities of decolonising data as part of determining the way forward for South Africans during COVID-19.

When exploring colonialism, what emerges is that apartheid, data colonialism, and racial capitalism in South Africa are resurfacing themes of dispossession. Although the scale of violence may differ across these aspects, the interrelationship between colonialism and capitalism remains intact. Inexpensive labour is thus replaced with inexpensive data, and privacy regarding data mimics the disregard for privacy during the colonial and apartheid era (Piotrowski, 2019; Mariotti & Fourie, 2014; Ogura, 1996; Terreblanche, 1994). In this way, present-day social life is transformed into data relations as humans connect on social platforms. In data relations, people are subject to data colonialism, not through violence but instead through force and deception. This force exhibits itself as a compulsory need to download applications in the continued pursuit of social relations (Couldry & Mejias, 2019a). The deception lies in general ignorance when downloading applications, as people are not always aware of the hidden details associated with the download. The existing desire for social relations forms a dependency that exposes people to being exploited, often without them realising fully what has happened. More importantly, these data relations and social platforms prolong racist, sexist, and class violence without the physical element (Couldry & Mejias, 2019a). Therefore, racism and sexism can target vulnerable groups, subjecting them to oppression in the digital space, which has an effect in the real world. Having said this, the question is what the decolonising[4] of data would resemble in South Africa. This question is essentially how people could resist data colonialism in South Africa. Is this resistance against data colonialism even possible? What would such resistance involve? These questions are part of the decolonising exercise, as the colonial nature of data must receive recognition before anyone can begin to speak of decolonising data.

Recognising how data may be used for dispossession purposes in society, specifically during the COVID-19 pandemic, is part of decolonising data. This process includes the identification of data on social platforms as not merely information, but information that may be used for deception and influence (Couldry & Mejias,

2019a). To limit the influence that data relations and data colonialism may have on an individual, it is necessary to engage in decolonising the mind (Wa Thiong'o, 1986). Since the mind takes in all the information displayed on a technological device, it becomes crucial to separate the aspects relating to misinformation and disinformation and prevent them from becoming accepted as the truth. This requires a consciousness of the strategies imposed on technological sites to succeed in exploitation and deception (Couldry & Mejias, 2019a). The mind is subjected to psychological and social damage inflicted by data colonialism, and for this reason it is necessary for the mind to be liberated from the damaging effect of knowledge in the digital space. Delineating fiction from truth in the digital realm can be a taxing undertaking, yet if people do not engage their minds and consider the truth of the information provided on social platforms, they will fall victim to misinformation and disinformation (Couldry & Mejias, 2019a; Maldonado-Torres, 2016; Wa Thiong'o, 1986).

When giving consideration to decolonising data and eliminating data colonialism, individuals are forced to become aware of the intentional politics of separation and how coloniality and apartheid (Piotrowski, 2019; Mariotti & Fourie, 2014; Ogura, 1996; Terreblanche, 1994) are filtering through the current management of COVID-19 in South Africa. The separation between the classes, which was historically influenced by the separation of race groups into different areas, has become visible during the COVID-19 pandemic. This separation has caused the unequal division of resources and access to health facilities, which has left Black people at a perpetual disadvantage (Piotrowski, 2019; Mariotti & Fourie, 2014; Ogura, 1996; Terreblanche, 1994). In addition, the COVID-19 pandemic divides the digitally knowledgeable from the digitally disadvantaged, the sick from the healthy, and the poor from the wealthy. All of these divisions are underpinned by coloniality and capitalism (Couldry & Mejias, 2019a). The aforementioned divisions serve to privilege some and disadvantage others, thereby creating a system of disempowerment. It is because of these divisions that the members of society are cautioned against binary thinking and advised instead to challenge these categories in society, including the treatment of those in the categories deemed problematic (Maldonado-Torres, 2016).

Decolonising data is necessary for freedom and autonomy, which are being threatened by the rise of technology and the dependency created through data relations. Just as colonialism and apartheid were fought collectively, the collective should similarly fight data colonialism (Couldry & Mejias, 2019a). This brings to mind ubuntu, which is best captured as "a person is a person because of or through others" (Moloketi, 2009: 243; Tutu, 2004: 25–26) The concept of *ubuntu*, which promotes the connectedness of persons, shows how people may unite in solidarity against the data colonialism that affects all of humankind (Moloketi, 2009; Tutu, 2004). Although digital space and social platforms are used for socialising and connecting, people need to be aware of the dangers associated with digital space. Consequently it is useful to think of digital space as a producer and a product; therefore it is important to consider both when using such spaces (Li & Zhou, 2018; Harvey, 2006).

Moreover, people as users of data similarly become producers in the digital space while also being produced by this space (Li & Zhou, 2018; Harvey, 2006). When the role of people as users in a digital space is given consideration, the awareness of their active involvement in this space emerges, including how they actively desire to re-create a space that is conducive to achieving connectedness and not separation (Li & Zhou, 2018; Harvey, 2006). Although the digital space may alter the way people relate to one another, they need to be vigilant not to become socialised into behaviours that are oppressive to others and encourage an ideology of separateness in South Africa.

These thoughts on decolonising data colonialism are by no means exhaustive and require much further research and interrogation. This chapter merely seeks to present the necessity for and advocate the call to decolonise the digital space, and in so doing preventing a new form of colonisation.

Conclusion

This chapter put forward the argument that data contains some tenets of appropriation that were present in historical colonialism. Knowledge in the digital world holds power and influence. However, private data organisations and corporations that are linked with colonial superpowers such as China and the United States have been engaging in unbalanced and disproportionate acts that allow ownership in the data collection process. Ownership pertains to those organisations that have rights to the hardware and software that process the data. The element of capitalism is evident when viewing the economic dominance that arises from large-scale processing of data and the data analysis capabilities that establish a degree of power in the social quantification of human functioning.

COVID-19 and the measures imposed to curb its spread have advanced the transition to a digital approach in performing labour activities. Data-processing power and the value extracted from individuals sharing information in cyberspace have paved the way for new frameworks for understanding the factors "community" and "datafication". The book The Costs of Connection, by Couldry and Mejias (2019b), has dramatically influenced the manner in which colonialism offers insight into the "geographically" located neo-colonial tool, namely "data", in social contexts.

In South Africa, there are still remnants of the colonial past that have facilitated the fragmentation of communities and the unequal distribution of economic resources. Time and labour are facets of value that are extracted because of human functionality in a digital space. In a nation such as South Africa, which is still exhibiting a great digital divide, aspects of power and knowledge influence that are derived from data dominance still elude the majority to a large degree. The robust nature of internet activity in South Africa may ultimately mean that individuals who have limited access to a digital environment are excluded. The movement towards new labour, created because of an advanced digital domain, will of necessity imply that some workers will be excluded from an evolving market. The authors warn against how Black people may be particularly vulnerable to racial capitalism as COVID-19 threatens to reproduce social and economic inequalities. The exploration of data colonialism in South Africa is essential for advancing decoloniality and imperative for a social justice praxis.

Notes

1 Athlone is a residential area predominately inhabited by "Coloured" people in Cape Town, South Africa.
2 "Racial profiling is a crime prevention and detection method, used by police officers, which takes racial identity into account to select and investigate suspects" (Zack, 2015, p. 47).
3 Couldry and Mejias (2019b) refer to data colonialism. In addition, see Mezzadra and Neilson (2017) on the extraction of data in social society.
4 Decolonising refers to the breakdown of colonial structures of power, knowledge, and being.

Acknowledgements

This work is based on the research supported by the National Institute for The Humanities and Social Sciences (NIHSS).

References

Access Partnership. 2020. *Facial Recognition Technology: A Primer*. www.accesspartnership.com/cms/wp-content/uploads/2020/09/AP-Primer-to-Facial-RecognitionTechnology (accessed 7 December 2020).
Angeles, L. 2013. On the causes of the African slave trade. *Kyklos*, 66(1): 1–26.
Blount, K. 2017. Body worn cameras with facial recognition technology: When it constitutes a search. *Criminal Law Practitioner*, 3(4). https://digitalcommons.wcl.american.edu/clp/vol3/iss4/4
Buzan, B. 1991. *People, States and Fear: An Agenda for International Security Studies in the Post-Cold War Era*. Essex: Longman.
Carter, P. L. 2009. Geography, race, and quantification. *The Professional Geographer*, 61(4): 465–480.
Cavelty, M. and Wegner, A. 2020. Cyber security meets security politics: complex technology, fragmented politics, and networked science. *Contemporary Security Policy*, 41(1): 5–32.
Chowdhury, N. H., Adam, M. T. P. and Skinner, G. 2019. The impact of time pressure on cybersecurity behaviour: A systematic literature review. *Behaviour & Information Technology*. https://doi.org/10.1080/0144929X.2019.1583769
Cilliers, J. 2020. *Africa First: Igniting a Growth Revolution*. Johannesburg: Jonathan Ball Publishers.
Cook, A. and Kemeny, T. 2017. The economic geography of immigrant diversity: Disparate impacts and new directions. *Geography Compass*, 11: 1–23.
Couldry, N. and Mejias, U. 2018. Data colonialism: Rethinking big data's relation to the contemporary subject. *Television and New Media* Vol 33 (4): 1– 14. DOI:10.1177/1527476418796632.
Couldry, N. and Mejias, U. A. 2019a. Making data colonialism liveable: How might data's social order be regulated. *Internet Policy Review*, 8(2). https://doi.org/10.14763/2019.2.1411.

Couldry, N. and Mejias, U. A. 2019b. *The Costs of Connection. How Data is Colonizing Human Life and Appropriating it for Capitalism.* Redwood City, CA: Stanford University Press.

Davenport, C., Soule, S. A. and Armstrong, D. A. 2011. Protesting while black: The differential policing of American activism, 1960 to 1990. *American Sociological Review*, 76(1): 152–178. https://doi.org/10.1177/0003122410395370

Encyclopaedia Britannica. 2018. Trojan Horse. *Encyclopaedia Britannica.* www.britannica.com/topic/Trojanhorse (accessed 16 November 2020).

Evans, C. M., Egan, J. R. and Hall, I. 2018. Pneumonic plague in Johannesburg, South Africa, 1904. *Emerging Infectious Diseases*, 24(1): 95–102. doi: 10.3201/eid2401.161817

Gandy, O. 2019. The algorithm made me do it! Predictive policing, cameras, social media and affective assessment. *Conference Proceeding.* https://web.asc.upenn.edu/usr/ogandy/Algorithm.pdf (accessed 5 December 2020).

González, F., Yu, Y., Figueroa, A., López, C. and Aragon, C. 2019. Global reactions to the Cambridge analytica scandal: A cross-language social media study. In *Companion Proceedings of the 2019 World Wide Web Conference Association for Computing Machinery, San Francisco, USA*, 799–806. New York: ACM. https://doi.org/10.1145/3308560.3316456

Harvey, D. 2006. Space as a keyword. In *David Harvey: A Critical Reader*, edited by Noel Castree and Gregory Dimitri, pp. 70–93. Hoboken: Blackwell Publishing Ltd.

Isaacs-Martin, W. 2018. Minority identities and negative attitudes toward immigrants: Prejudice and spatial difference amongst the Coloured population in South Africa. *African Review*, 10(1): 41–57.

Johnson, A. 2020. *Coronavirus: Africans Accuse Europeans of 'Coronising' Continent: Commentators in Africa Note a 'Reversal of Roles' with European Countries Struggling to Contain Pandemic.* www.middleeasteye.net/news/coronavirus-africans-accuse-europeans-coronising-continent (accessed 1 December 2020).

Koen, H. S. 2017. *Predictive Policing in an Endangered Species Context: Combating Rhino Poaching in the Kruger National Park.* (Master's dissertation). Pretoria: University of Pretoria.

Kumar, S., Saravanakumar, K. and Deepa, K. 2016. On privacy and security in social media – A comprehensive study. *Procedia Computer Science*, 78: 114–119.

Lapaire, J. R. 2018. Why content matters. Zuckerberg, vox media and the Cambridge analytica data leak. *ANTARES: Letras e Humanidades*, 10(20): 88–110.

Lever, A. 2016. Racial profiling and the political philosophy of race. In *The Oxford Handbook of the Philosophy of Race*, edited by N. Zack, pp. 425–435. New York: Oxford University Press.

Li, X. and Zhou, S. 2018. The trialectics of spatiality: The labelling of a historical area of Beijing. *Sustainability*, 10(2018): 1–20.

Lyon, D. 2014. Surveillance, Snowden, and big data: Capacities, consequences, critique. *Big Data & Society*, 1: 1–13.

Maldonado-Torres, N. 2016. Outline of ten theses of coloniality and decoloniality. Franz Fanon Foundation. http://franzfanonfoundation (accessed 8 November 2020).

Marivate, V. and Combrink, H. 2020. Use of available data to inform the covid-19 outbreak in South Africa: A case study. *Data Science Journal*, 19(1): 19. http://doi.org/10.5334/dsj-2020-019

Mariotti, M. and Fourie, J. 2014. The economics of apartheid: An introduction. *Economic History of Developing Regions*, 29(2): 113–125.

Meijer, A. and Wessels, M. 2019. Predictive policing: Review of benefits and drawbacks. *International Journal of Public Administration*, 42(12): 1031–1039. https://doi.org/10.1080/01900692.2019.1575664

Meiring, T., Kannemeyer, C. and Potgieter, E. 2018. *The Gap between Rich and Poor: South African Society's Biggest Divide Depends on Where You Think You Fit in.* Cape Town: SALDRU, UCT (SALDRU). Working Paper No 220. https://www.opensaldru.uct.ac.za/bitstream/handle/11090/901/2018_220_Saldruwp.pdf

Mezzadra, S. and Neilson, B. 2017. On the multiple frontiers of extraction: Excavating contemporary capitalism. *Cultural Studies*, 31(2–3): 185–204. doi: 10.1080/09502386.2017.1303425

Moloketi, G. R. 2009. Towards a common understanding of corruption in Africa. *Public Policy and Administration*, 24(3): 331–338.

Ogura, M. 1996. Urbanization and apartheid in South Africa: Influx controls and their abolition. *The Developing Economies*, XXXIV–4: 402–422.

Oliver, E. and Oliver, W. H. 2017. The colonisation of South Africa: A unique case. *Theological Studies*, 73(3): 8. https://doi.org/10.4102/hts.v73i3.4498

Pandya, P. 2013. The enemy (The intruder's Genesis). In *Computer and Information Security Handbook* (3rd ed.), edited by J. R. Vacca, pp. E45–E56. Burlington: Morgan Kaufmann.

Pillay, A. L. and Barnes, B. R. 2020. Psychology and COVID-19: Impacts, themes and way forward. *South African Journal of Psychology*, 50(2): 148–153. https://doi.org/10.1177/0081246320937684

Piotrowski, A. 2019. Colonialism, apartheid and democracy: South Africa's historical implications on the land reform debate. *Journal of Interdisciplinary Undergraduate Research*, 11(4): 53–71.

Rossi, A. 2018. How the snowden revelations saved the EU general data protection regulation. *The International Spectator*, 53(4): 95–11.

Sambumbu, S. 2010. Reading visual representations of 'Ndabeni' in the public realms. *Kronos*, 36(1): 184–206.

Savić, D. 2020. COVID-19 and work from home: Digital transformation of the workforce. *The Grey Journal*, 16(2): 101–104.

Schneier, B. 2015. *Data and Goliath*. New York: Norton.

Seacom. 2020. *How Much Internet Traffic in South Africa Has Increased Due to the Coronavirus.* https://seacom.co.za/media-centre/how-much-internet-traffic-south-africa-has-increasedRdue-coronavirus/ (accessed 5 December 2020).

Shan, T., Chen, S., Sanderson, C. and Lovell, B. C. 2007. Towards robust face recognition for intelligent-CCTV based surveillance using one gallery image; *INSERT Day and Month 2007 IEEE Conference on Advanced Video and Signal Based Surveillance*; dates from to. *Place: Publisher*, 470–475. https://doi.org/10.1109/AVSS.2007.4425356

Solomon, S. 2018. Cambridge Analytica played roles in multiple African Elections, March 22. www.voanews.com/africa/cambridge-analytica-played-roles-multiple-african-elections (accessed 1 December 2020).

Song, P. X., Wang, L., Zhou, Y., He, J., Zhum, B., Wang, F., Tang, L. and Eisenberg, M. 2020. An epidemiological forecast model and software assessing interventions on COVID-19 epidemic in China. *MedRxiv*. https://doi.org/10.1101/2020.02.29.20029421 (accessed 2 December 2020).

Soucie, J. M. 2012. Public health surveillance and data collection: General principles and impact on haemophilia care. *Journal of Haematology*, 17(1): 144–146. https://doi.org/10.1179/102453312X13336169156537

South African Government Gazette. 2002. *Disaster Management Act: Amendment of Regulations Issued in Terms of Section 27(2). Vol 657. No 11062.* Pretoria: Government Printer.

South African History Online. 2020. *The Trojan Horse Massacre: 15 October 1985.* www.sahistory.org.za/dated-event/trojan-horse-massacre (accessed 7 December 2020).

Staunton, C., Swanepoel, C. and Labuschaigne, M. 2020. Between a rock and a hard place: COVID-19 and South Africa's response. *Journal of Law and the Biosciences*, 7(1): 1–12. https://doi.org/10.1093/jlb/lsaa052

Stuurman, Z. 2020. Police brutality in South Africa exposed once again. *Mail & Guardian*, 28 August. https://mg.co.za/opinion/2020-08-28-police-brutality-in-south-africa-exposed-once-again/ (accessed 5 December 2020).

Sun, R., Wei, W., Minhui, X., Gareth, T., Seyit, C. and Damith, R. 2020. *Vetting Security and Privacy of Global COVID-19 Contact Tracing Applications*. www.researchgate.net/publication/342352381_Vetting_Security_and_Privacy_of_Global_COVID-19_Contact_Tracing_Applications (accessed 12 December 2020).

Terreblanche, S. J. 1994. From white supremacy and racial capitalism towards a sustainable system of democratic capitalism – a structural analysis. Transit (SJT33), University of Stellenbosch. www.ekon.sun.ac.za/sampieterreblanche/wp-content/uploads/2018/04/SJT-1994-From-white-supremacy-to-racial-capitalism.pdf (accessed 28 October 2020).

Trippe, K. 2020. *Pandemic Policing: South Africa's Most Vulnerable Face a Sharp Increase in Police-Related Brutality*. www.atlanticcouncil.org/blogs/africasource/pandemic-policing-south-africas-most-vulnerable-face-a-sharp-increase-in-police-related-brutality/ (accessed 2 December 2020).

Trotter, H. 2019. Trauma and memory: The impact of apartheid-era removals on coloured identity in Cape Town. In *Burden by Race: Coloured Identities in Southern Africa*, edited by M. Adhikari, pp. 49–78. Cape Town: UCT Press.

Tutu, D. 2004. *God Has a Dream: A Vision of Hope for Our Future*. London: Rider.

Van Der Spuy, A. 2020. Colonising ourselves? An introduction to data colonialism. *Research ICT Africa*. https://researchictafrica.net/2020/03/23/colonising-ourselves-an-introduction-to-data-colonialism/ (accessed 2 December 2020).

Van Dijk, J. 2014. *The Culture of Connectivity*. Oxford: Oxford University Press.

Vreÿ, F. and Solomon, H. 2020. COVID-19 as a security threat: Some initial perspectives. Security Institute for Governance and Leadership in Africa. *Research Brief*, 7.

Wa Thiong'o, N. 1986. *Decolonizing the Mind: The Politics of Language in African Literature*. Harare: Zimbabwe Publishing House.

Wang, J. 2018. *Carceral Capitalism*. Semiotext Intervention Series. Los Angeles, CA: Semiotext(e) Press.

West, S. M. 2019. Data capitalism: redefining the logics of surveillance and privacy. *Business & Society*, 58(1): 20–41. https://doi.org/10.1177/0007650317718185

Zack, N. (2015). White privilege and black rights: the injustice of U.S. police racial profiling and homicide. Rowman & Littlefield.

8

OCCUPATIONAL HEALTH IN THE MINING INDUSTRY OF SOUTH AFRICA AND THE COVID-19 PANDEMIC

Robert Maseko

Introduction

This chapter attempts to highlight the plight of Black mineworkers in South Africa and their continued death and struggle with occupational health diseases. The main argument is that mineworkers are treated as the dispensable other. Death is an everyday experience for Black mineworkers, who toil underground for many years and after contracting diseases such as silicosis and tuberculosis are usually dumped by their employers and later released from their duties with little or no form of compensation. Using the available literature and in-depth interviews with affected mineworkers, this chapter aims to expose the tendency to use and abuse these mineworkers by the mines, and most of the times regulations are not followed to protect mineworkers from contracting these diseases. This research was conducted partly from the period of 2014 to 2016 in Rustenburg with mineworkers working for the then Anglo Platinum, Khuseleka Mine (now Sibanye Stillwater) and those working for Aquarius Mine K5. The two mines are located within a kilometre of each other on the north-western side of the city of Rustenburg, North West Province. All in all, 33 mineworkers from Khuseleka mine and 6 mineworkers from Aquarius Mine were interviewed with regard to their health and working conditions. Most of these workers have since been decimated by diseases such as tuberculosis (TB), silicosis, HIV, and COVID-19. These mineworkers were either staying at Jabula Hostel which is located near Khuseleka Mine and Sondela, an informal settlement, or they stayed in rented accommodations in and around Sondela. The study did not interview any female mineworkers. To protect their identity in this chapter, I will use their interview information as anonymous, except those of the union leaders, who gave consent to use their real names. The rest of the chapter is structured as follows: the first part delves deep into the history of silicosis in the South African mines and

DOI: 10.4324/9781003415121-8

their continued exposure to diseases while working underground. I also introduce the concepts of the zone of non-being as a theoretical lens in understanding the plight of mineworkers in South Africa; the second part deals with the vast literature on the process of compensating affected mineworkers as well as the COVID-19 pandemic. It introduces the landmark silicosis ruling which found in favour of the affected mineworkers to be compensated for the diseases acquired while working underground; in doing so the chapter focuses on the recent COVID-19 pandemic and how it has affected the process of compensating mineworkers.

The history of silicosis in the South African mines

The history of mining in South Africa is a history of injustice, invasion, appropriation, and forced labour. Mineworkers were sourced from all over the region and coerced into working in dangerous mining conditions for little or no pay in what Bernard Magubane would describe as being paid a slave wage. The colour bar, which was designed to protect certain jobs from white people, had ensured that both Black and white mineworkers were involved in the underground work activities (for example, Black mineworkers were rock drillers and lashers while white mineworkers were underground supervisors and explosive experts) (Katz, 1999), thereby both racial groups were exposed to occupational lung diseases. The system of segregation continued to have a negative impact on the majority Black mineworkers, who continued to die in large numbers and in particular when the apartheid government took over in 1948. Occupational ill-health and injuries at work have had a huge impact on the total gross domestic product (GDP) and some indirect costs of livelihood loss, income, and social trauma (Harmanus, 2007). By the early 20th century most white miners had taken up supervisory roles as a result of the racist state policies while dusty underground jobs had been given solely to Black migrant workers, thus silicosis has been more prevalent in Black mineworkers while TB and pneumonia were more common in white workers (Ehrlich, 2012). More than half of the mineworkers in South Africa were from the neighbouring countries such as Mozambique and Lesotho; furthermore, the present mineworkers are outnumbered by former mineworkers (Ibid). This means that compensation for mineworkers affected by silicosis and TB is likely to be much higher.

According to Meel (2003) for the first 15 years after the discovery of gold deposits in the Witwatersrand, silicosis was unknown until mineworkers started dying in large numbers. The sad part is that as this was happening, sick mineworkers from some countries of what is now known as the Southern African Community Development (SADC) region were compensated with money for a train ticket back home. However, in 1911, the Miners' Phthisis Allowance Act (Act No. 34 of 1911) was promulgated, a legislation designed to compensate mineworkers who were affected by silicosis. Compensation for miners came at a time when the gold mines in Johannesburg were hardest hit by occupational lung diseases (Katz, 1994). The compensation for Black mineworkers was marred by racial injustices and biases;

there was little emphasis on issues of safety and health of mineworkers as companies were obsessed with making a profit and disregarding issues of human rights and dignity (Maloka, 1996). Most Black mineworkers were kept in barrack-like compound housing where movement was controlled (Mamdani, 2017). Designed to control African labour, the compound system became a death trap for many Africans seeking a better life, or a means of survival, on the mines. Many succumbed to curable diseases due to the inhumane conditions in the compounds with diseases such as TB, asbestosis, and silicosis (arising from working the mines) being the main killers of Black mineworkers (McCulloch 2003, 2012; Maloka, 1996). According to Ehrlich (2012) if a disease was confirmed, white mineworkers were entitled to a full pension pay-out, while for Black mineworkers only a once-off payment was granted without even considering the severity of the disease. The 1911 Act was succeeded by the Occupational Diseases in Mines and Works, Act No. 78 of 1973 (ODMWA). In 1973 Black mineworkers (who relied on substandard medical equipment of the mine where many cases were missed) had their contracts terminated if silicosis was confirmed, while the same law never applied to white mineworkers who had access to medical examinations at a state medical bureau in Johannesburg.

The Commission of Inquiry into Mine Safety and Health found out in 1995 that the exposure to respiratory diseases for those working underground has not changed for more than half a century (Harmanus, 2007). In his study of former mineworkers in the Transkei Region (now Eastern Cape), Meel (2003) found out that 78% of the retrenched and retired mineworkers were in a poor state of health and living in abject poverty, unable to secure any form of employment anywhere and as a result most of them ended up committing suicide. Studies of former mineworkers in the Eastern Cape and Botswana indicated that about 20% of former Black mineworkers had contacted silicosis, painting a grim picture of the prevalence of the disease in the mining industry in South Africa (Churchyard et al., 2004). To add on to that, former president of South Africa, Nelson Mandela in his book *Long Walk to Freedom* highlighted the fact that the youngest men from the region of Transkei who went to look for employment in the mines came back sick, and their families could not even recognise them on their return. This is what Nelson Mandela had to say about the lives of the young people that were destroyed in the mines:

> They will cough their lives out deep in the bowels of the white man's mines, destroying their health, never seeing the sun; so that the white man can live a life of unequalled prosperity. . . . I was not destined to work in the gold mines on the Reef. The regent had often told me, "It is not for you to spend your life mining the white man's gold, never knowing how to write your name".
>
> *(Mandela, 1994:30)*

All this points to the fact that former mineworkers had underlying health conditions acquired while working in underground tunnels for many years. In actual fact, Molaka (1996) argues that during the period of the late 1800s to early 1900s the mines were a source and spread of diseases to Southern African rural communities. However, because of the lack of investment in the health system and prevention of diseases like silicosis, white mineworkers were also victims of this silicosis, as most of them died from this incurable disease (Katz, 1994). According to Katz, focus was given to the white mineworkers who were dying as a result of silicosis in large numbers. Owing to high death rates through diseases such as silicosis and TB in the mines among white mineworkers, the white government designed legislation which specified compensation to those affected. Black people were totally excluded from this, but the post-apartheid government amended the legislation (the ODMWA in 2002) to include Black people and thereby remove the racist clauses in the act. Cases recorded for silicosis for Black mineworkers was always very low as compared to white miners, as the white government was never concerned about the plight of Black mineworkers (McCulloch, 2009).

The ODMWA was enacted in 2002 to undo the injustices of the past and to prevent more Black mineworkers from contracting occupational lung diseases. More than 100 years since the gold mines were hit by the occupational lung disease, Black mineworkers continue to die in the mining industry (Ehrlich, 2012). The ODMWA was thus meant to consolidate and amend laws regarding compensation of certain diseases to people who have contracted the diseases while working in the mines. Different organisations had worked together to formulate and bring the amended legislation to fruition and to ensure that victims were compensated and silicosis eradicated, and these included the World Health Organization (WHO), International Labour Organisation (ILO), National Mineworkers union (NUM), the Chamber of Mines, and the Ministry of Health (McCulloch, 2009).

The main goal of the act was to compensate those diagnosed with the diseases listed in the legislation as well as those who got injured at work. In the case of death or illness, Chapter 6 of the act stipulates and gives clarity on the beneficiaries entitled to compensation (including the family of the deceased) and the terms and conditions of compensation. All evaluations and diagnosis of silicosis must first be done through the Medical Bureau for Occupational Diseases (MBOD) based in Braamfontein, Johannesburg (Roberts, 2009). However, according to Section 99 of the act, no person shall be compensated due to diseases not listed. This is problematic given the existence of the AIDS pandemic, where even the slightest effects of undetected silicosis and TB can result in fatal consequences for mineworkers living with HIV and AIDS. The act gives an opportunity for mineworkers to sue the mining company for compensation if found with any of the listed diseases, but the majority of the mineworkers are unable to fight within the law as they are illiterate and the compensation procedures are complicated, and they are often unwilling to pursue such cases (Roberts, 2009; Banyini, 2012). It is also the case that silicosis can resurface 20 years after the miner has returned home to his rural area, and to seek compensation after so many years is exceedingly difficult (even if the name of the mine is remembered).

Despite the promulgation of the ODMWA, deaths as a result of diseases continue to interrupt mining activities, cause considerable harm and distress to mineworkers and their families, and generally create economic and social strain within the mining industry. In a parliamentary debate on 19 June 2014, Minister of Health Dr Aaron Motsoaledi gave shocking statistical figures about the high number of mine deaths in post-apartheid South African mines as a result of TB and silicosis (Department of Health, 2014; *City Press* 20 January 2014). Motsoaledi acknowledged the importance of the mining industry in the South African economy as well as the 500,000 mineworkers employed in the mines across the country. Because the country was facing a serious challenge from the HIV pandemic, 80% of those living with the disease were killed by TB, and mineworkers were the hardest hit by this (Department of Health, 2014). Some of the facts in his speech are as follows:

- There are about 41,810 TB cases in the mines every year in South Africa.
- There are 500,000 mineworkers, 230,000 of their partners, and 700,000 of their children directly affected.
- Twenty per cent of these partners and children are in Lesotho, Mozambique, and Swaziland.
- A total of 59,400 orphans are currently in care as a result of TB-related deaths in the mining sector.
- A total of 9.6 million workdays are lost each year to TB.
- In 2009, 167 fatalities occurred in the mining sector due to mining accidents; 24,590 cases of TB in the mining sector led 1,598 TB fatalities also in 2009.
- The gold mines are the most affected, with 80 fatalities due to mining accidents in 2009.
- There were 17,591 TB cases in the mining sector alone which led to 1,143 deaths. Hence, for every death of a miner due to accidents, there are nine deaths due to TB.
- The stability of the mining industry in the country is dependent on the ability to fight TB.

(Dr Aaron Motsoaledi, Department of Health, 19 June 2014:01–05)

From this speech by Dr Aaron Motsoaledi, it is evident that death in the mines, particularly for Black mineworkers, is still a reality. The ODMWA was designed to ensure that mineworkers are paid compensation, but companies are often unwilling to pay such that workers no longer seek a diagnosis, and current cases of diseases are covered up by companies to avoid payments. Giving evidence to the Leon Commission of Inquiry in 1994, Senzeni Zokwana, the then president of NUM, reiterated that the mine work underground was difficult and risky, and he also highlighted the problem of power and control contributed to these dangers. He suggested that workers should be given rights to choose to work or refuse when there was danger to their health (McCulloch, 2012). This statement is critical as it reflects questions of the rights and dignity of mineworkers as well as coloniality of being, something which is addressed later in this chapter.

Social death in the zone of non-being

Human beings can actually die a social death before their biological death (Mulkay & Ernst, 1991), and this is true in the case of Black mineworkers in South Africa. Our ability to recognise others determines the existence or non-existence of social death in any society (Sweeting & Gilhooly, 1997). The concept of "non-persons" (people who are otherwise invisibilised and marginalised by the system and from the social world) by Goffman cited in Mulkay and Ernst (1991) as the major cause of social death is similar to the concept of the zone of non-being by Frantz Fanon whereby some people are inferiorised and considered less human than others. Those who are considered to be non-persons and socially reside in the zone of non-being experience death every day, and similarly death has been normalised in this space and also contributes negatively to social life. Sweeting and Gilhooly (1997) argued that personhood makes life more valuable, and those who have lost their personhood are perceived to be as "good as dead" because they have lost all characteristics of humanity.

For Gordon (2007), to re-humanise Black people, there is a need for an elaborate process of mediation on what it means to be "human". On the people who "do not exist" as argued by Fanon, Gordon states "I look into the lived-reality of people hidden in plain sight – people who are submerged and, as a consequence, supposedly 'do not exist'. It has always struck me as odd that people could be invisible while standing right before us" (Gordon, 2007: 107). In his psychoanalytical studies, Fanon was able to link the plight of Black people (the people who do not exist) to their past traumatic experiences that continue to affect their present lives. Most people end up suffering from psychological trauma, poor mental health, post-traumatic stress and develop psychiatric problems mainly because of their past experiences. The experiences of the colonial past, poverty, death, diseases, hunger, and desperation have a negative impact socially and on the health of the affected people, and thus many of the majority poor die a social death before their biological death. Abdul Jan-Mohamed talks about "death-bound subjectivity", and these are people living with the possibility of death; according to Gordon (2007:11) "it means witnessing concrete instances of arbitrary death and social practice that demonstrate that one group of people's lives are less valuable than others' to the point of their not being considered to be really people at all".

Most mineworkers die in social violence where they are denied good health and most of the times are subjected to inhuman working conditions where their fate is sealed. Death-bound subjectivities hop from one social condition to the other, for example, what happens to the mineworker when he comes to the mine and what happens when he leaves the mine. The psychological trauma and mental trauma have an impact socially and on the health of mineworkers – this is a form of social violence whereby mineworkers are denied good health and are exploited for profits. During the COVID-19 pandemic, health and social institutions, including the living conditions of those marginalised, remain far from the expected standard to prevent the spread of the virus. The lack of proper housing for mineworkers, the absence of tap water, and the absence of social distancing in the informal settlements of South Africa all make increased conditions of vulnerability for Black mineworkers to COVID-19, TB, and silicosis.

The continued exposure to silicosis

In this section I discuss how systematically mineworkers are exposed to silicosis and TB by intentionally disregarding safety of mineworkers. The working lives of these (and the other dismissed) workers is nothing short of hellish. At K5 shaft, the early morning shift is supposed to report at the outside gate of the mine at 5:00 am and then proceed to the changing rooms where workers are expected to change and put on the mining gear. The mining gear and other work-related equipment are very heavy to carry to the underground work site. The chairperson of the Association of Mineworkers and Construction Union (AMCU) (based at Anglo-Platinum Khuseleka Shaft) Siphamandla Makhanya spoke about this more generally, saying that mineworkers work under very difficult conditions. They have to wear mining gear which weighs more than 5 kilograms for the whole day without any time to rest or eat; in addition, they carry a drilling machine which weighs up to 60 or 65 kg. Returning to the work schedule at K5, mineworkers are expected to report to the second gate by 5:30 am.

Those who come just minutes after 5:30 am at the second gate, despite having reported by 5:00 am at the main gate, are recorded by mine management as "half shift or short shift", meaning that they will earn half-salary for the work done for the day. At the second gate, mineworkers are expected to wait in a waiting area (often in freezing temperatures) for more than two hours, as those from the night shift come out between 6.30 am and 7:00 am. When the night shift is cleared, early morning underground blasting takes place. Then those in the early morning shift have to wait for the "dust to settle down" before going underground at 8:00 am to start their actual work. During this time dust and smoke still fill the underground tunnels, and workers are forced to go inside with little visibility. Among those going inside are the so-called "half shift or short shift" who reported at the gate soon after 5:30 am. Mineworkers then toil in dust- and smoke-filled tunnels non-stop until 4:00 pm or in some cases until 6:00 pm including those who are said to be "half shift or short shift". The mineworkers, once underground, also have to work sometimes within very narrow tunnels in a bending and kneeling position and under very hot and moist conditions. According to the workers, the mine has one of the highest cases of TB and silicosis in South Africa, and the majority of these cases are not reported or put on official record. For Magubane (2007) this shows that Black people are the "dispensable other", while for Maldonado-Torres (2007:255) this demonstrates "killability and rapeability" predicated on killing, torture, and rape which are inscribed on Black bodies.

Condemned to death

In the mining industry in South Africa diseases amongst mineworkers are particularly prevalent and in a sense have devastated the workforce. This is no less true at Khuseleka. Hence, those interviewed for this research, including union leaders, stress that one of the key challenges facing the mining industry today is the high number of disease-related deaths that are threatening to bring the "golden goose" to its knees. This was also highlighted by Minister of Health Dr Aaron Motsoaledi on 19 June 2014 in a parliamentary debate.

Silicosis and TB remain the biggest killers of mineworkers since colonial and apartheid times, as articulated by Van Onselen (1976), Jeeves (1985), Allen (1992), and many others. However, what makes these deaths particularly disturbing is that the prevalence of silicosis remains concealed by the mines as well as by hospitals and medical doctors, who become part of a system that hides the truth on the scale of the diseases so that mines can avoid compensating their mineworkers. In this respect, it should be noted that death or ill-health as a result of silicosis is payable or can be compensated for. By and large, mining companies are unwilling to pay for such ill-health or death of mineworkers occurring as a result of work at the mines. And because at Anglo Platinum Mine, as elsewhere, Black people are the ones working underground, silicosis and TB will continue to be the biggest killers among Black mineworkers.

During an interview with the AMCU chairperson of education at Anglo Platinum Khuseleka Mine on the prevalence of diseases among mineworkers, Mr Lazarus Khoza reiterated that as many as 300 workers per day are given day off by doctors, and the figure could be more as some workers do not disclose their sickness to the mine; he further argued that most of these diseases are as a result of some diseases acquired outside the mine such as HIV and AIDS (Khoza, L. personal communication, 3 September 2014).

This statement from Mr Khoza is a gruesome revelation of how serious the question of health is among the mineworkers, and this of course threatens the viability of the mining industry, as most of these diseases are acquired while working in the mines. The branch chairperson of Anglo Platinum Khuseleka Mine, Siphamandla Makhanya, argues that most workers have TB as a result of their working conditions. "The majority of these workers, because of their working conditions, they end up having what they call spinal code TB or they have TB, which is not TB in actual fact but silicosis in real sense" (Makhanya, S. personal interview 3 September 2014). Unlike in previous years when silicosis and TB killed Black mineworkers together with white miners (Allen, 1992; Leger, 1992; Maloka, 1996), today these diseases have become a Black man's disease mainly because there are now few underground white mineworkers in the country and most notably at Anglo Platinum

Khuseleka Mine. Most white mineworkers at Anglo Platinum, if not holding supervisory positions, go underground to check on work being done and then soon return to the surface. One anonymous mineworker said that blast smoke is the major killer of underground mineworkers, because workers are forced to go underground even before the smoke has been cleared (Anonymous, personal communication, 18 August 2014).

All mineworkers interviewed in this research spoke about the high prevalence of suffering from ill-health and linked this explicitly to the conditions under which they work underground. And when they become sick, they accuse the mine of ending their work contract without compensation. Another low-level miner said, "When you are sick the mine is losing because you are no longer productive'" (Anonymous, personal communication, 18 August 2014). The mine does not want to keep sick people on its payroll, and this is when the relationship between a miner and the mine becomes most tense. In this respect, a miner who is a rock driller gave an example of a cow and when it can no longer work for its owner the owner will have to "dump" it. He was referring to the way in which Anglo Platinum treats its Black workers when they are no longer productive because of ill-health (Anonymous, personal communication, 18 August 2014).

A 55-year-old mineworker argues further that when one becomes sick, "The mine behaves as if they have never known you before despite having worked for them for many years" (Anonymous, personal communication, 18 August 2014). McCulloch (2012) argues that the majority of mineworkers who are diagnosed with silicosis and TB are sent home by mine management to die, and those who seem fit can develop signs of silicosis years after they have left the mine (for example, due to retirement). Usually when Black mineworkers are no longer wanted by the mines, they will go back to their rural homelands where they will die in poverty, as argued by Meel (2003) in his research on the suicide rate among former mineworkers. However, because of fear of losing their jobs if they reveal that they are sick, most mineworkers remain silent and continue working, and this only serves to accelerate the disease. Another mineworker emphasised that because of their already marginalised economic condition because of low wages, they will not disclose their ill-health for fear of losing their job and being sent back home. Most interviewed miners made claims that if a mineworker continues complaining about being sick, he risks having what they called a "bad record" from the perspective of mine management. The mine will then send such a worker to a medical board so that he can be certified unfit to work and be relieved of his duties. And from there, they say, "The mine is done with you", meaning the mine will never try to follow up and monitor the circumstances of the mineworker after being discharged from work.

Some mineworkers argued that the moment one declares that he is not feeling well, this is the time when the mine (Anglo Platinum) "wants you out of their premises as soon as possible". For some of these mineworkers, the moment one declares his sickness, "everything changes from that day; the mine cannot keep you anymore" (Anonymous, personal communication, 18 August 2014). Most interviewed workers stated that they fear being sent to the medical board because no one has ever come back to work after being sent to this board; in short all have been certified unfit and sent home.

The articulation by branch chairperson of AMCU, Mr Makhanya, on this matter is very significant, as he noted that diseases such as silicosis which are subject to compensation by the mine are under-diagnosed deliberately to protect the mines from paying the workers the required compensation. He also notes the existence of a syndicate inclusive of mine management and the medical system which props up this condition of coloniality by concealing silicosis as the killer disease for Black mineworkers at Anglo Platinum (Makhanya, S. personal interview 3 September 2014). Hence, to remove all responsibility for the ill-health of mineworkers, the mine reconstructs the health problem as emanating from outside the mine and therefore washes its hands clean of all guilt.

However, even if the disease emanated from outside work conditions, the mine cannot disclaim all responsibility. Indeed, not all diseases arise through underground work, because some diseases are acquired from where mineworkers stay, notably under the inhumane conditions in terms of the shack accommodations at the informal settlement at Sondela, as described earlier. Sondela is a key site of accommodation for mineworkers because the wages paid by the mine are inadequate for obtaining decent accommodation. But even problems exist at the Jabula Hostel on the mine site. Some mineworkers argued that the food offered at Jabula Hostel makes them sick, but they are forced to eat it, as they are not allowed to buy food and cook for themselves. One mineworker who is originally from Botswana, who stayed in the hostel for many years before moving out to Sondela where he rents a shack, says he was sick for many years until the doctors found out that the food he was eating at Jabula Hostel was making him sick. His good health has returned because he now can buy food of his choice rather than being forced to eat food at the Jabula dining hall. At the same time, he notes that Sondela has its own health problems: it is filthier than at Jabula Hostel, the shacks are in a bad condition, there is significant overpopulation, and he stays close to the dumpsite where pollution is high.

For the chairperson of AMCU, Mr Makhanya, the laws pertaining to worker health that were enacted soon after independence (during the reign of NUM on the mines) need to be changed. He says the existing legislation, at least at the level of implementation and enforcement, are not in favour of Black mineworkers today, particularly given that they are the ones affected most by diseases such as silicosis and TB. According to him, the existing legislation is reminiscent of "apartheid laws" whereby once a mineworker has been diagnosed with silicosis or TB, he is immediately removed from his job, instead of them (the mine) removing him from underground work and maybe trying to find lighter surface work for him. Instead, Black mineworkers are simply discarded like an obsolete and un-repairable machine would be scrapped and written off, which is the type of point raised by Magubane (2007) in delineating the fundamentals of coloniality.

Landmark silicosis ruling for mineworkers

The landmark silicosis ruling for mineworkers was a court action by the affected mineworkers taken against mining giants who included African Rainbow Minerals, Anglo American SA, AngloGold Ashanti, Gold Fields, Harmony, and Sibanye-Stillwater. One of the lighter sides of the South African litigation process for the affected mineworkers is that it involved various stakeholders such as trade unions, the government, the mining companies, non-governmental organisations (NGOs), politicians, and the media (Meeran, 2003). On 3 May 2018, the court ruled in favour of the mineworkers who had taken a legal route to seek compensation for those who were affected by silicosis. The ruling came as a reprieve to many affected former and present mineworkers who for years have worked in the mines and contacted silicosis and TB and never been compensated, with the majority of mineworkers dying in extreme poverty, having been abandoned by the same mines they worked for. According to the court ruling, four categories of claimants were identified (from Class 1 silicosis to Class 4), and this also included the families of the dead miners if proven that indeed the mineworker died as a result of silicosis or TB that he contracted while working in a mine. The amount of money varies with each category of claimant, ranging from 10,000 Rands to 500,000 Rands (Kotze, 2020). The Tshiamiso Trust Fund was to be formed to oversee the administration of the fund, the distribution of the funds, and the tracking down of claimants. On the basis of all this, the silicosis legal claim is argued to be far bigger than any other claim in the global history of industrial disasters. For example, it is said to be bigger than the Chernobyl and the Fukushima nuclear disasters as well as the Bhopal chemical disaster in India in terms of those injured (Bateman, 2012).

However, the settlement of the silicosis and TB class action suit has also been criticised by many. For example, some have accused the companies of lacking committeemen in the establishment of the trust that should oversee the administration of the distribution of the funds to the affected mineworkers and the tracking down of the affected mineworkers dating back to those who worked in the mines in early 1960s. Two years after the landmark ruling, there is still no payment made to the affected mineworkers (James, 2020). Without a functioning trust, the dream of compensating mineworkers remains in limbo and more and more affected mineworkers continue to die, and some have argued that this is the intention of the mining companies that are responsible for these payments – to continue delaying so that less money can be paid to dead miners rather than when they are alive. The court order did not give specific time frames for the formation of the trust, thereby allowing mining companies to use this as an opportunity to deny compensation for more mineworkers when they are still alive. In short there is a lack of commitment from the mining companies in establishing a functioning trust to kick-start the process of compensating affected miners. A statement released by the Justice for Miners Campaign (J4C) group in July 2020 expressed concern over the suspension of lung function tests due to COVID-19 that are required by the affected miners to undergo in order to ascertain those who qualify for compensation, which means there is going to be further delays in the process of compensation (Stent, 202). According to some, it can take from 18 months to five years for payments to start rolling out, but also this is dependent on the attitude, obligations, and willingness of the mining companies (Bateman, 2012). With all the silicosis underlining conditions, most affected miners are likely to die from COVID-19 and risk losing all the benefits.

COVID-19, tuberculosis, and silicosis

COVID-19, TB, and silicosis are all respiratory diseases with usually similar symptoms, and all require speedy diagnostics (Karim & Karim, 2020). Mineworkers in South Africa are housed in squalid and crowded housing environments where social distancing is impossible with shared toilets and tap facilities, and hand washing and self-isolation are virtually impossible (Boffa et al., 2020). Many mineworkers have chronic conditions which compromise their immune system, making them vulnerable to COVID-19. Studies have shown that those with drug-resistant TB are at increased risk from COVID-19 (Boffa et al., 2020). COVID-19 cases are increasing in South Africa, with a new COVID-19 strain discovered in 2021 which has spread all over the world and in particular Southern Africa. This phenomenon is likely to be disastrous to those already living in poverty and already infected with silicosis, HIV, and TB from the years of working in the mines. More so, COVID-19 is believed to be spreading much faster in closed spaces such as inside a room, and this means that those working in underground tunnels are more likely to get infected than those working in outside environments. COVID-19 mitigation measures are more difficult in underground mining than in an open cast mining environment (Jowitt, 2020). In short, underground mining is a fertile ground for breeding and spreading COVID-19, TB, and silicosis.

COVID-19 infections have a high chance of interrupting TB and silicosis treatment, and this may result in loss of life of many infected mineworkers in South Africa and the neighbouring countries that provide labour in South African mines. A combination of TB and COVID-19 is likely to result in poor treatment outcome and deadly results (Boffa et al., 2020). Now as the country is reeling from a collapsing health system as a result of COVID-19 infections, priority has shifted to combat the spread of COVID-19 over TB and silicosis, with previous existing resources being redirected to combat the spread of coronavirus (Karim & Karim, 2020). As such, more silicosis and TB patients are likely to die from this policy shift. Hard lockdowns during the coronavirus pandemic have resulted in many mineworkers returning to their rural homes, where health facilities are not equipped or do not exist, and this will also result in more devastating consequences for those living with HIV, TB, and silicosis. Africa, and South Africa in particular, remain one of the areas hardest hit by HIV and TB.

The post-COVID mining order

Diagnostic and testing centres for TB and silicosis have been greatly affected during lockdowns, and this means the identification of those in need of compensation has stalled and more affected miners are likely to die (Karim & Karim, 2020). The closing of country borders and reduction in public centres have also made things difficult for those located in the rural communities and those in the neighbouring countries like Mozambique, Lesotho, Zimbabwe, Malawi, and Botswana. Laboratory testing for TB, HIV, and silicosis is now used for COVID-19 testing (Karim & Karim, 2020). About 28,000 HIV community health care workers were redeployed to fight the coronavirus pandemic, and this means that most HIV programmes are paralyzed (Ibid). Lack of personal protective equipment (PPE) and staff shortages for front-line workers to fight the pandemic in mostly rural clinics in South Africa have seriously affected the spread of the virus and the prevention of death (Kim, 2020). The South African Minerals Council has urged commitment among mining companies to fight the spread of COVID-19 among mineworkers (Murray, 2020).

The COVID-19 pandemic has collapsed some countries' economies at a scale never seen before, and the mining industry has not been spared either. Globally, the mining industry has halted operations or is operating at 50% capacity as the price of minerals has slumped to the lowest it has ever been as a result of reduced demand for the mining products (Laing, 2020). By the end of 2020 the mining industry in South Africa had dropped to about 8% to 10% in its production as a result of the pandemic (Murray, 2020). Unlike other mines that are located in remote areas with smaller populations, mines in South Africa are usually located near densely populated communities, which makes it easy for the virus to spread. Now that the vaccine for COVID-19 has been found, priority is given to the front-line workers and mineworkers will not be a priority, and this might also have disastrous consequences. What this means is that the process of identifying TB- and silicosis-infected mineworkers is going to be seriously affected as all operations have been halted. More and more mineworkers will continue to die mainly because priority is now given to fight the spread of COVID-19 and, on the other hand, the unwillingness of the mining companies to speed up the process of compensation for the affected mineworkers. Today mines are encouraged to invest in digital technologies in combating the spread of COVID-19 (Atif et al., 2020) with efforts to fight TB and silicosis halted.

According to David Rees, emeritus professor of occupational medicine and epidemiology at the University of the Witwatersrand, infections among mine workers reflect the conditions in the communities where they reside. More infections should be expected in the coming months, he added, "What is happening in the mines is to be expected. It is not extraordinary, given that infections in the country are currently on the rise" (Khumalo, 2020). The conditions under which Black mineworkers live make it difficult to fight infections diseases such as COVID-19 and

TB. Just like Professor Rees, the chairperson of the then Anglo Platinum Khuseleka Mine (now Sibanye Stillwater) Siphamandla Makhanya, said the living and housing conditions of Black mineworkers in communities around the mines represent their working conditions underground. In other words, the fight against the COVID-19 pandemic, both at the place of production (at work) and the place of reproduction (at home), should be a policy priority for both government and mining companies. However, the NUM has blamed the rise in infections to the mines for failing to adhere to the rules and regulations to combat the spread of COVID-19.For example, they claim that while the government recommended shutting down mining operations during lockdown, some mines continued their operations as normal, and during this time COVID-19 protocols were not followed, exposing mineworkers to the virus; they argue that mines are chasing profits ahead of the lives of mineworkers (Khumalo, 2020).

As the country lockdowns continue, this will also have a serious effect on the mineworkers, as well as former mineworkers based outside the country who qualify to be compensated for diseases acquired while working in South African mines. They will be unable to cross the borders to be tested for silicosis in order to receive their compensation in testing centres located in the country. On 25 June 2020 Bloomberg News reported that the platinum mines in South Africa were facing a serious problem of returning thousands of skilled mineworkers who were stranded in neighbouring Mozambique, Swaziland, Lesotho, and Botswana during the COVID-19 national lockdown (Felix Njini, 2020). By the look of things from the evidence given by the mineworkers in the previous sections, mines will continue to relieve and retrench those mineworkers who became sick as a result of infectious diseases acquired while working underground. There is a high chance that mines will continue resisting the payment to and compensation for affected mineworkers, and they might argue that COVID-19 had devastating consequences on their finances. COVID-19 might be used to stall any claims for compensation by former and present mineworkers, and more and sick mineworkers will continue to die in poverty. Jowitt (2020) argued that the COVID-19 pandemic is likely to fuel clashes between the government and the mining companies mainly because the government is likely to pass laws that compel companies to shut down operations while the companies might feel obliged to continue with operations. In this case the government might try to force companies to adhere to the judgment of the high court which ruled in favour of compensating mineworkers affected with TB and silicosis, while companies might argue that the pandemic has actually put them in a state of bankruptcy.

What does it mean to be a Black mineworker?

To be a mineworker means being confronted with the possibility of social death, only to return home to face biological death in poverty. Thus, though officially the government after apartheid no longer blocks or inhibits urban migration (for instance, through pass laws), the prospects of a permanent urban presence for mineworkers from the zone of non-being is thwarted through the ongoing exploitation of mine-workers by mining companies. For Moodie (1994) the life of a Black mineworker was in his rural homeland, where he was expected to return after his contract in the mine had expired and he was expected to reproduce to keep the supply chain of cheap labour going in the mines.

A semi-proletarianised young Black man had no choice but to work in the mines, on white farms, and increasingly in manufacturing industries as a survival strategy; here they encountered face-to-face the reality of oppression and segregation (Magubane, 1983, Seekings & Nattrass, 2005, Magubane, 2007). Likewise, in an article written by Thabo Mbeki in 1971 titled "Why I Joined the Communist Party," Mbeki recalls seeing men coming from the mines very thin and sick to the extent that even their children could not recognise them after toiling for several years in the mines (Roberts, 2009). These men died in poverty without any compensation. Now during the time of the COVID-19 pandemic, mineworkers are likely to be affected the most mainly because their social conditions have not changed for many years.

Being a miner also has a clear racial (Black), gendered (male), and class (working class) identity and dimension, and it is marked by brutal conditions of existence. All affected workers in this study were Black and from poor rural backgrounds. Black migrant workers in South Africa, both rural migrants and foreign migrants, likewise grapple with such hellish conditions in the mining industry. And in this darker side of Western modernity (or in the zone of non-being), tensions and conflicts are often not resolved by managing differences through negotiations, but by means of coercion (Fanon, 1968, Santos, 2007). Even in the case of contemporary South Africa, where formal racism as existed under apartheid has been abolished, the non-white subject continues to experience daily indignities. These "outsiders" are regularly portrayed as "a problem", if not "the problem", for instance, by failing to assimilate into the prevailing hegemonic order (in the core) or by refusing to abide by constitutional and formalistic procedures in their protests and struggles in the periphery (William Du Bois cited in Gordon, 2007). These "wretched of the earth" (in Fanon's terms) stand accused of all sorts of despicable acts, such as crime, environmental destruction, and overcrowding.

Conclusion

From the beginning of the 20th century, mine owners knew about the dangers of contracting silicosis in the mines, but no action was taken to prevent mineworkers from getting the disease. Despite the possibility that with proper dust control measures underground silicosis can be prevented, many mines have not complied with these regulations, exposing thousands of Black mineworkers to silicosis and TB. The housing and living conditions of mineworkers have left them exposed to TB, silicosis, and now the COVID-19 pandemic. The pandemic has respected no borders – all Southern African countries are affected – and this puts former and present mineworkers in a dire situation. In the litigation case against the mines organised by the affected former mineworkers, Nkala reiterated how there was complete silence on the dangers of contracting silicosis (Field, 2019). However, despite full knowledge of the presence of the disease, even the post-apartheid mine system still forces mineworkers to work in dangerous environments even after the complaints, like in the case of Aquarius mineworkers. The situation is now exacerbated by the unlikely combination of the triple diseases, namely HIV, TB, and silicosis, that have devastated the Black communities, which has generated some debate as to whether or not these three are subject to be compensated for because of the manner in which TB and HIV can be contracted. Some argue that they can also be contracted outside the mining environment; hence the mines cannot solely be blamed for the prevalence of these diseases (Bateman, 2012). Now, the COVID-19 pandemic presents another dilemma in the politics of compensating mineworkers, and this dilemma is likely to create tensions between the government and the mines. However, the possibilities of new questions are likely to surface: is COVID-19 a compensable disease if contracted in the underground working environment?

The dispensability of a Black miner's life in the platinum belt is vividly evident, as is the ferocity of capital. In large part all this remains unchallenged, even by the government, such that the Black mineworker is sacrificed in order to maintain coloniality and wealth in contemporary South Africa. In light of what happened at Aquarius Platinum Mine, I conclude that a Black mineworker is still not regarded as a human being, because his dignity and ontological density have been stripped. It seems, then, that the coloniality of power and being thrives in the platinum industry despite the end of the colonial condition in 1994. This, in the end, is the only conclusion that can be drawn when the voices of Black miners are given space and openly heard and a complete decolonisation of the political economy occurs. By and large the fight against the deadly COVID-19 pandemic will require a coordinated effort among the global countries, and for now the closing of international borders seems to have little and less effect. In this age of globalisation and modernity characterised by connectivity among humanity, a pandemic like this has once again highlighted how some political leaders want to believe in isolating themselves from other people. A fight for this pandemic does not require blaming other countries, blaming other races and cultures, but a collective effort among people globally. The COVID-19 pandemic has no respect for international and artificially created borders.

References

Allen, V. L. 1992. *The History of Black Mineworkers in South Africa: The Techniques of Resistance 1871–1948* (Vol. 1). Yorkshire: The Moor Press.

Atif, I., Cawood, F. T. and Mahboob, M. A. 2020. The role of digital technologies that could be applied for prescreening in the mining industry during the COVID-19 pandemic. *Transactions of the Indian National Academy of Engineering*, 5(4): 663–674.

Banyini, A. V. 2012. *Utilisation of Autopsy Services for Posthumous Monetary Compensation Among Black Mine Workers in South Africa*. (PhD Thesis). Johannesburg: University of Witwatersrand.

Bateman, C. 2012. Silicosis: 10 000 gold miners getting set to sue. *SAMJ: South African Medical Journal*, 102(6): 338–340.

Boffa, J., Mhlaba, T., Sulis, G., Moyo, S., Sifumba, Z., Pai, M. and Daftary, A. 2020. COVID-19 and tuberculosis in South Africa: A dangerous combination. *SAMJ: South African Medical Journal*, 110(5): 1–2.

Churchyard, G. J., Ehrlich, R., Pemba, L., Dekker, K., Vermeijs, M., White, N. and Myers, J. 2004. Silicosis prevalence and exposure-response relations in South African goldminers. *Occupational and Environmental Medicine*, 61(10): 811–816.

Department of Health. 2014. *Debate on the State of the Nation Address Minister of Health, Dr Aaron Motsoaledi*, 19 June. www.gov.za/speeches/view.php?sid=46162 (accessed 13 October 2014).

Ehrlich, R. 2012. A century of miners' compensation in South Africa. *American Journal of Industrial Medicine*, 55(6): 560–569.

Fanon, F. 1968. *Black Skin, White Masks, Trans, Charles Lam Markmann*. New York: Grove Press.

Felix Njini. 2020. Virus-hit South African mines battle to return workers. *Bloomberg News*, 25 June. www.bloomberg.com/news/articles/2020-06-25/virus-hit-south-african-miners-battle-red-tape-to-return-workers (accessed 8 January 2021).

Field, T. L. 2019. Exacting silicosis justice through the class action mechanism. *Mineral Economics*, 32(2): 213–221.

Gordon, L. R. 2007. Through the hellish zone of nonbeing, Thinking through fanon, disaster, and the damned of the earth. *Human Architecture: Journal of the Sociology of Self-Knowledge*, (5): 5–11.

Harmanus, M. A. 2007. Occupational health and safety in mining – status, new developments and concerns. *The Journal of The Southern African Institute of Mining and Metallurgy*, 107: 531–538.

James, M. 2020. Mining output in South Africa set to drop this year due to coronavirus. *NS Energy Business*, 29 May. www.nsenergybusiness.com/news/south-africa-mining-coronavirus/ (accessed 8 January 2021).

James, S. Two years after landmark silicosis settlement, no-one has been paid. *TimesLive News*, 21 July. www.timeslive.co.za/news/south-africa/2020-07-21-two-years-after-landmark-silicosis-settlement-no-one-has-been-paid/ (accessed 21 July 2020).

Jeeves, A. H. 1985. Migrant labour in South Africa's mining economy. In *The Struggle for the Gold mines' Labour Supply*, pp. 1820–1920. Johannesburg: Wits University Press.

Jowitt, S. M. 2020. COVID-19 and the global mining industry. *SEG Discovery*, 122: 33–41.

Karim, Q. A. and Karim, S. S. A. 2020. COVID-19 affects HIV and tuberculosis care. *Science*, 369(6502): 366–368.

Katz, E. N. 1994. *The White Death: Silicosis on the Witwatersrand Gold Mines 1886–1910*. Johannesburg: Witwatersrand University Press Publications.

Katz, E. N. 1999. Revisiting the origins of the industrial colour bar in the Witwatersrand gold mining industry, 1891–1899. *Journal of Southern African Studies*, 25(1): 73–97.

Khumalo, S. 2020. Nealy 3000 cororavirus cases at mines, with platinum workers bearing the brunt. *News24*, 6 July 2020. www.news24.com/fin24/companies/mining/nearly-3-000-coronavirus-cases-at-mines-with-platinum-workers-bearing-the-brunt-20200706 (accessed 8 January 2021).

Kim, H. 2020. The daily battle of rural nurses on South Africa's COVID-19 frontline. *Reuters News*, 6 October. www.reuters.com/article/us-health-coronavirus-safrica-nurses-trf/the-daily-battle-of-rural-nurses-on-south-africas-covid-19-frontline-idUSKBN26R1LB (accessed 8 January 2021).

Kotze, C. 2020. Silicosis settlement: First claimant pay outs expected in Q2. *Mining Indaba*, 2 April. www.miningreview.com/gold/silicosis-settlement-first-claimant-pay-outs-expected-in-q2-2020/ (accessed 21 July 2020).

Laing, T. 2020. The economic impact of the Coronavirus 2019 (COVID-2019): Implications for the mining industry. *The Extractive Industries and Society*, 7(2): 580–582.

Leger, J. P. 1992. Occupational diseases in South African mines: A neglected epidemic? *South African Medical Journal*, 81: 197–201.

Magubane, B. 1983. Imperialism and the making of the South African working class, Review work(s): Contemporary marxism, No. 6, Proletarianization and class struggle in Africa. *Social Justice/Global Options*, 19–56.

Magubane, B. 2007. *Race and the Construction of the Dispensable Other*. Pretoria: UniSA Press.

Maldonado-Torres, N. 2007. On the coloniality of being. *Cultural Studies*, 21(2–3): 240–270.

Maloka, T. 1996. 'White death' and 'Africa disease': Silicosis on the witwatersrand gold mines. *South African Historical Journal*, 34(1): 249–254.

Mamdani, M. 2017. *Citizen and Subject: Contemporary Africa and the Legacy of Late Colonialism*. Johannesburg: Wits University Press.

Mandela, N. R. 1994. *Long Walk to Freedom, Volume 2, 1962–1994*. London: Little Brown.

McCulloch, J. 2003. Women mining asbestos in South Africa, 1893–1980. *Journal of Southern African Studies*, 29(2): 413–432.

McCulloch, J. 2009. Counting the cost: Gold mining and occupational diseases in contemporary South Africa, *African Affairs*, 108/43(1): 221–240.

McCulloch, J. 2012. *South Africa's Gold Mines & the Politics of Silicosis*. Johannesburg: Jacana.

Meel, B. 2003. Suicide among former mineworkers in the sub region of Transkei, South Africa. *Archives of Suicide Research*, 7(3): 287–292.

Meeran, R. 2003. Cape Plc: South African mineworkers' quest for justice. *International Journal of Occupational and Environmental Health*, 9(3): 218–229.

Moodie, T. D. 1994. *Going for Gold: Men, Mines and Migration' with Vivienne Ndatshe*. Berkeley: University of California Press.

Mulkay, M. and Ernst, J. 1991. The changing profile of social death. *European Journal of Sociology/Archives Européennes de Sociologie/EuropäischesArchivfürSoziologie*, 32(1): 172–196.

Murray, E. J. 2020. Epidemiology's time of need: COVID-19 calls for epidemic-related economies. *Journal of Economic Perspective*, 34(4): 105–120.

Occupational Diseases in Mines and Works Act 78 of 1973 (ODMWA). www.ilo.org/wcmsp5/groups/public/--- . . . /wcms_190734.pdf (accessed 17 October 2014).

Roberts, J. 2009. *The Hidden Epidemic Amongst Former Miners: Silicosis, Tuberculosis and the Occupational Diseases in mines and Works Act in Eastern Cape, South Africa*. Department of health, Health Systems Trust. chrome-extension://efaidnbmnnnibpcajpcglclefindmkaj/https://www.equinetafrica.org/sites/default/files/uploads/documents/ROBehs01092009.pdf (accessed 19 May 2023).

Roberts, R. S. 2007. *Fit to Govern: The Native Intelligence of Thabo Mbeki*. STE Publishers.

Santos, B. S. 2007. Beyond abyssal thinking: From global line to ecologies of knowledge. *Review*, XXX(1): 45–89.

Seekings, J. and Nattrass, N. 2005. *Class, Race, and Inequality in South Africa*. New Haven: Yale University Press.

Sweeting, H. and Gilhooly, M. 1997. Dementia and the phenomenon of social death. *Sociology of Health & Illness*, 19(1): 93–11.

Van Onselen, C. 1976. *Chibaro: African Mine Labour in Southern Rhodesia 1900–1933*. Johannesburg: Ravan Press.

9

"ON EST PAS DE COBAYES"

Congolese migrants and health transnationalism in the COVID-19 moment[1]

Leon Mwamba Tshimpaka
and Christopher Changwe Nshimbi

Introduction

The 2019 coronavirus disease (COVID-19) broke out in Wuhan, China, and rapidly spread to other parts of the world, especially Europe and North America. The disease was slow to spread to and within Africa, with the first case only recorded in Egypt on 14 February 2020. The World Health Organization (WHO) eventually declared the disease a pandemic. This was on 11 March 2020, about a month after Africa recorded the first case. The declaration came almost three months after the authorities in China had, on 31 December 2019, informed the WHO about a pneumonia of unknown cause and without cure or vaccine. The recommended solutions then, therefore, were social and included *inter alia* maintaining physical distances (or social distancing) between people of at least one metre, washing hands with soap or alcohol-based sanitisers, and wearing masks in public.

For governments and health professionals, emphasis in executing their public health mandate was placed on tracing contacts of people who had tested positive for the disease, isolating infected people, and administering intensive medical care to patients who exhibited severe symptoms. Countries also enforced strict measures that restricted human mobility such as closures of nation-state borders and imposition of curfews. This was done in order to contain and slow down the spread of the disease. Accordingly, when the first case of the disease was detected in Kinshasa in the Democratic Republic of the Congo (DRC) on 10 March 2020,

[1] This study was partially funded by the Migration and Inclusive Societies (MIS) visiting fellowship program at Luxembourg University's Faculty of Humanity, Education, and Social Sciences (FHESC) in 2023.

DOI: 10.4324/9781003415121-9

the country's president, Felix Tshisekedi, declared a national state of disaster. This was after he had established a presidential task force and a multi-sector COVID-19 response unit. The DRC, of course, built on its experience in dealing with Ebola to improve on its national response to COVID-19. In the absence of a known cure, however, misinformation and myths about COVID-19, possible solutions, and measures to stop the spread circulated in local communities and on the internet and social media.

This chapter examines the messages of Europe- and North America–based Congolese migrants and their engagements with people and communities back home on issues regarding COVID-19. The chapter builds on the notions of transnationalism and public health governance to examine how the migrants influenced people and communities back home. It does this by attempting to respond to the question: what kind of COVID-19–related messages do Congolese migrants engage with/in and send to people and communities back home? How are those messages conveyed? That is, what channels or media do they use to convey the messages? How do the targets or recipients of the messages back home respond? Why do Congolese migrants engage people and communities back home on such issues? Based on the analysis of data drawn in response to these questions and explained in the methods and approaches section, the chapter argues that the Congolese diaspora engages in health transnationalism in order to influence people's "health behaviour" and the governance of public health back home. They do this in a quest to promote well-being and improve the Congolese public health sector.

Methods and approaches to understanding transnationalism and public health governance in DRC

The chapter is based on a qualitative research design that deploys a content analysis approach. It addresses the questions raised and meets its objective by analysing content including Congolese migrant messages that relate to COVID-19. The content is drawn from social media, including platforms like YouTube and WhatsApp, as well as broadcast media talk shows. Migrants generally use these platforms and channels to communicate and share experiences in the diaspora with people back home. As further discussed in the chapter, some of the specific information analysed includes narratives and experiences of migrants' recovery from COVID-19 through the application of indigenous methods of treatment. The chapter thus unpacks some COVID-19–related messages of Congolese migrants sent to people back home and considers the types of delivery channels and/or media that the migrants use to convey their messages. It then examines the domestic response to the migrants' messages and goes on to discuss the migrants' engagement with people and communities back home. In addition to analysis of media content, the chapter also extensively reviews the literature on migration and health governance to inform the analysis.

Transnationalism and public health governance: some conceptual considerations

The Congolese diaspora maintains strong ties and a love for the motherland (Tshimpaka, 2020, 2021). The strong tie and love of country of origin relate to transnationalism in international migration studies. Migrants manifest/express transnationalism while abroad in various forms, including through socio-economic remittances, preference for and consumption of homeland food, listening to homeland music, and practising homeland culture and intercontinental citizenship (Bauböck, 2003, 2006; Bauböck & Faist, 2010; Tshimpaka, 2020). We posit in this chapter that, in the COVID-19 moment, the Congolese diaspora in Europe and North American expressed its tie and love of country of origin in a way that sought to influence people's public health and public health governance.

Health transnationalism

We view health transnationalism as a wide range of international activities and practices that are related to public health and developed by migrants who have strong ties with their country of origin. Health transnationalism can also be viewed as social relations through health-related activities beyond national borders (Njoya, 2009; Perullo, 2008). The health transnational activities and practices of migrants are mostly aimed at promoting public health in the homeland. We take cognisance of the possibility that good health may not necessarily be the absence of disease and physical disability but also includes the absence of environmental pollution as well as emotional and psychological imbalances. We therefore agree with the WHO's definition of health as "a state of a complete physical, mental, and social well-being and not merely the absence of disease or infirmity" (WHO, 1948: 1). Moreover, health is "a resource for everyday life, not the objective of living [. . . but . . .] a positive concept emphasizing social and personal resources, as well as physical capacities" (WHO, 1948; Ryff & Singer, 1998; Smith et al., 2006). With the help of these definitions, we can broaden the understanding of health beyond that conception that it relates to illness and infirmity. Actually, our conception fits well with the way that the Southern African Development Community (SADC) Health Protocol perceives health in its preamble. It asserts that "it is aware that a healthy population is a prerequisite for sustainable human development and increased productivity in Member States" (SADC, 1999:1). Euro-American–based Congolese migrants seem to be very concerned with the precarity in and of the public health sector back home. This drives them to send messages that aim to influence people's health behaviour and the public health governance system in the COVID-19 moment.

Without digressing into debates on the conceptualisation and theorisation of transnationalism, we acknowledge that it can be perceived in multi-dimensional ways in different contexts that might be cultural, political, economic, religious, or medical. Transnationalism focuses on migrants' networks and their agency in different spheres of life that tie them in culture, economics, politics, and health that are all associated with their country of origin (Østergaard-Nielsen, 2003, Bauböck, 2006; Bauböck & Faist, 2010). The notion can be viewed as part of political, environmental, cultural, and socio-economic remittances made by migrants to their home countries. In this regard, we agree with Schiller et al. (1992: ix) who define transnationalism as "the processes by which immigrants build social fields that link together their country of origin and their country of settlement". The migrants develop and maintain multiple relationships including religious, political, economic, familial, organisational, and social that tie them to their countries of origin (Vertovec, 2003; Tshimpaka, 2020, 2021). Migrants act, decide, feel, and develop identities in social networks through which they simultaneously connect to two or more societies (Schiller et al., 1992; Bauböck & Faist, 2010). The international connections may take the form of overlapping or interconnected socio-cultural, political, economic, and health practices that link host countries with the homeland (Lima, 2010; Tedeschi et al., 2020). We thus conceptualise health transnationalism as the international social practices and activities of migrants within the public health sector that link them to people, communities, and government back home in ways that seek to influence behaviour and public health governance. Physical mobility that enables migration, virtual mobility, and virtual tools such as information communication and technologies (ICTs) and information on disease and the quality of public health in both sending and receiving countries are essential to international participation in health transnationalism. This is the context in which, in the COVID-19 moment, Congolese migrants were concerned that the government back home was not prepared to deal with the pandemic and sought to intervene.

Public health governance

Public health governance constitutes the way in which government, the private sector, and civil society respectively and in total deploy efforts that cover the breadth and nature of wide-ranging legal and regulatory approaches to protect, promote, and restore physical and mental well-being for the majority of a population (Coggon et al., 2017). It is the system of principles and related rules that a society uses to manage its population's health. This is the sense in which the SADC Health Protocol defines it as "the effort of society to protect, promote and restore the people's health through health-related activities in order to reduce the amount of diseases, premature death, and reduce discomfort and disability in the population" (SADC, 1999: 2). Similarly, Verweij and Dawson (2007: 21) view public health as the "collective interventions that aim to promote and protect the health of the public". We too adopt this view of public health governance in this chapter. It is an effort that is not necessarily the sole responsibility of the state but is collective, involving both state and non-state actors, who then exhibit coordinated strategies, rules, and practices to ensure the protection, promotion, and restoration of a healthy population. Both state actors and non-state actors agree on the law, ethics, policies, and infrastructure that guide the regulation and coordination of the health of the whole of society through collective action (Munthe, 2008; Dawson, 2011, Dawson & Verweij, 2015). Therefore, public health governance is centred on three central elements, including a clear focus on the health of the majority of the population, prevention rather than cure, and collective effort (Dawson, 2011).

This is what the Congolese diaspora was concerned about in the COVID-19 moment in relation to the DRC – that it would not effectively deal with the pandemic. The diaspora is not alone in assuming this. The majority of Congolese at home are critical of the country's national health governance system. For its 80 million citizens, the DRC records only 406 hospitals and 8,126 clinics which are mainly owned by private and religious sectors (Reliefweb, 2020b). These health facilities are criticised because they are poorly equipped, inefficient, insufficiently funded, and lack accountability and transparency (Stasse et al., 2015, Trapido & Anaka, 2020). The general unavailability of enough medical centres across the country means that there are not enough quarantine sites to handle the COVID-19 health crisis. Some observers reproached the Congolese Ministry of Public Health for its lack of effective communication on the COVID-19 pandemic (Infobascongo, 2020). The government's handling of contact tracing and mass testing for COVID-19 was also criticised as ineffective and inefficient (Terrier, 2020). Thus, people allegedly felt abandoned and put in limbo with regard to the pandemic treatment and its regulation measures to control the contagion (Terrier, 2020; Radio Okapi, 2020). This is the situation that raised the concern of the Congolese diaspora in Europe and North America about the situation back home in DRC. The apparent crisis in handling COVID-19 prompted them to seek to intervene and influence public health governance back home through transnational health practices via, among other media, the internet. It should be pointed out, though, that the DRC is said to have built on lessons learned from responding to Ebola and applied them to tackling the COVID-19 pandemic (World Bank, 2020; Reliefweb, 2020b).

Congolese migrants and public response to the COVID-19 pandemic in DRC

The migration literature engages in debates on factors that drive many Africans to migrate to Europe and North America (Kirwin, 2018; Flahaux & De Haas, 2016). Some of these factors include poverty, economic hardships, persecution, civil wars, and political turmoil. For the DRC, such factors are also said to include poor governance, post-electoral crises, socio-economic disparities, diseases like Ebola, environmental disasters, and poor economic conditions (Montague, 2002, Kisangani, 2012, Versteeg et al., 2019, IOM, 2019, Tshimpaka, 2020, 2021). Whatever it is that drove them into migrating, Congolese migrants in Europe and North America engaged in health transnationalism with their home country in the COVID-19 moment, in reaction to what they perceived to be the poor handling and response to the pandemic by the government. To that end, they sent messages back home which seem to have had impacts on both the general public and the government, as the ensuing discussion demonstrates.

COVID-19 messages by Congolese migrants to their home country

The COVID-19 pandemic broke out when the DRC was fighting another pandemic – Ebola. Faced with two pandemics, the DRC certainly needed international aid to shore up its public health system. Yet, people in the Congolese diaspora sent messages about COVID-19 that largely contradicted and sought to provide alternative solutions to those recommended by the government and WHO. The migrants told people back home that COVID-19 did not exist in the DRC. They claimed that the virus could not withstand the heat and the weather in the DRC. The migrants went on to accuse government in the DRC of conniving with the WHO to vaccine people in exchange for money. In addition to this, migrants advised people back home to reject any vaccine trials until the vaccine was proven safe. They alleged that the vaccine had a microchip that would be injected in people in order to gather information about them (Reuters, 2020b; Kennedy, 2020). The migrants further asserted that the COVID-19 vaccine was part of a political strategy to control human minds and manipulate people's DNA. This would genetically manipulate recipients and constituted a silent crime against humanity (Kennedy, 2020). Anti-vaccine trial campaign videos that carried such messages as "*On est pas de Cobayes*[1]", featuring Congolese in the diaspora and some of whom included celebrities, went viral on social media (Reuters, 2020a). In this way, Congolese migrants advised people back home to be cautious with any medication and treatment provided by quarantine centres or hospitals. The WHO and other scientists dismissed the allegations made by the migrants in the diaspora as false (WHO, 2021). This, however, did not stop migrants from suggesting the use of indigenous remedies for people who opted to seek treatment for the disease. A proposed remedy, from an inexhaustive list, included daily steaming in which a user inhaled steam from a hot mixture of herbs including ginger, eucalyptus, citronella oil, lemon juice, onion, black pepper, and menthol vapour rub. Another included drinking human urine every morning for three days. Yet another remedy consisted of boosting one's immune system by drinking a hot mixture of honey, lemon juice, black pepper, ginger, and local herbs including one called *kongo-bololo*[2] (Africanews, 2020). Congolese migrants in Europe and North America also organised live and recorded talk shows on YouTube with diaspora-based Congolese medical doctors in which they discussed alternative methods of treating COVID-19 and myths about the vaccine. Interestingly, the migrants' messages seem to have had an impact back home, in the DRC.

Delivery channels of migrants' messages

Advancements in ICTs or "technologies of contact" in the late 20th century have facilitated transnationalism among migrants (Vertovec, 2009). Vertovec (2009) indicates that ICTs facilitate linkages between migrants and countries of origin through various tools including telephone, fax, email, satellite TV, and cheaper modes of travel. Added to this, digital tools that use social media platforms like YouTube, Facebook, WhatsApp, Twitter, and weblogs have increasingly become accessible and affordable. Migrants exploit them to communicate and keep in touch with people in their homelands (Lima, 2010). Likewise, Congolese migrants in Europe and North America use such online platforms, especially YouTube, WhatsApp, and Facebook, to communicate with people back home. Research on ICT use in the DRC actually shows that Facebook enjoys a high usage rate of 91% and WhatsApp 63%, and the services are provided by the country's four major telecommunications networks/internet service providers – Airtel, Orange, Tigo, and Vodacom (Target Sarl, 2015; GSMA Intelligence, 2019). The same research shows that demographically, WhatsApp seems to attract more women, who account for approximately 68% of users, while Facebook is more popular with men, who account for about 96% of users. The research further shows that young people in the age range between 25 and 35 years old constitute the majority of daily users of these online services (Target Sarl, 2015). The point to note here is that the online media platforms/applications like Facebook, WhatsApp, and YouTube that are popular with the Congolese diaspora and people back home are "cross-usable". A person who watches or comes across a message that is, say, broadcast on a YouTube channel such as Tele Tshangu1 can copy the link to that broadcast and paste it into their WhatsApp chat application and forward it to their contacts on WhatsApp. They can do the same on Facebook and other applications. Some users even edit video clips on their devices for various reasons and then forward or share the edited material with contacts/networks on their preferred platforms/applications.

Particular YouTube channels including Marius Muhunga TV, Barraud YouTube channel, Congo-France TV, Tele Tshangu1, Rhema TV, Mubenga TV, AparecoTV, Congo-Synthese, and Congo Mikili, are among the most popular fixed and/or mobile virtual TV stations that Congolese migrants use to beam messages back home (Mulongo, 2018; Tshimpaka, 2020). Europe- and North American–based Congolese migrants use these same media to send messages about COVID-19 with the aim of influencing the home country. Marius Muhunga TV in Washington, for example, carried an interview with a France-based Congolese migrant doctor, Jerome Munyangi, on 25 April 2020 in which Dr Munyangi alleged that an *Artemisia* plant-based protocol could cure COVID-19. Dr Munyangi also decried the hegemony of the WHO and alleged that the organisation was not pro-poor. He cited Madagascar President Andy Rajoelina's indigenous African herbal tonic and the WHO's refusal to endorse it among curative protocols for COVID-19 (see also, BBC News, 2020). Dr Munyangi called for the establishment of an African Health Organisation for Africans to own African public health (Marius Muhinga, TV, 2020). In May 2020, a YouTube video that featured late Tanzanian President John Pombe Magufuli went viral. In it, Magufuli questioned the reality of COVID-19 after non-human (goat, sheep, and papaya) samples tested positive for the disease in Tanzania. Magufuli's misgivings about the disease cemented Congolese migrants' claims and scepticism about the veracity of the COVID-19 pandemic (CGTN, 2020).

The Barraud YouTube channel aired another YouTube video that went viral on Facebook and WhatsApp and featured a French medical doctor, Didier Raoult, promoting hydroxychloroquine as an effective antidote and COVID-19 treatment. Dr Raoult, therefore, warned Africans not to take the COVID-19 vaccine. Dr Raoult further denounced pharmaceutical companies like Gilead Sciences and the WHO for threatening and prohibiting him from talking about hydroxychloroquine. He alleged that Gilead Sciences received a lot of money from the WHO to produce the COVID-19 vaccine (Barraud, 2020). Congolese migrants followed this up by posting short videos that supported Dr Raoult and the efficacy of hydroxychloroquine on Facebook and WhatsApp and targeted them to people in the DRC.

Response to migrants' messages in the DRC

The messages sent by people in the Congolese diaspora in Europe and North America have had an impact on both ordinary people and the government back home in the DRC.

Ordinary people's responses

The Congolese diaspora shared social media messages that raised scepticism of COVID-19 vaccine trials. Having been exposed to such videos as those of Dr Raoult and Dr Munyangi and "*On est pas de cobayes*", people opposed the DRC's participation in COVID-19 vaccine trials. Professor Dr Jean-Jacques Muyembe, head of the Congolese COVID-19 task team, had confirmed in a 3 April 2020 conference in Kinshasa that the DRC was ready to run COVID-19 vaccine trials in the country. In his own words, Professor Muyembe said, "We were chosen to do these tests". According to him, the vaccine would be produced in the United States, Canada, or China. Professor Muyembe further said, "We are candidates to do the tests here at home. Maybe around July, August we can already start to have clinical trials of this vaccine" (Ouest-France, 2020).[3] Professor Muyembe's announcement incited open resistance on the streets of the DRC and tension on social media. It simultaneously cemented the ongoing anti-vaccine trial messages conveyed by Congolese migrants to people back home, who refused to be used as guinea pigs in the trials. Mr Mohombi, a Swedish-Congolese musician, tweeted,

> Dear doctors, scientists and pharmaceutical empires. When you are done testing your COVID-19 vaccines on animals, before you even consider coming to try it on Africans, a people you have never shown consideration for, try it on yourself.
> *(Ouest-France, 2020)*[4]

Ordinary people, especially in the capital, Kinshasa, showed their scepticism of the reality and existence of COVID-19 in the DRC by not complying with government COVID-19 regulations. They further said it was impossible for them to observe such regulations as social distancing and curfews because they depended on informal trade and small-scale farming for survival. These livelihood activities, according to them, did not allow for the observation of COVID-19 regulations. Furthermore, people said they would rather risk their lives hustling outside and exposed to COVID-19 than die of hunger indoors. There was also the view, especially in the country's mega cities, that COVID-19 was a disease of the rich and *Mundele*,[5] or white-skinned people. Honourable Leon Nelemba Lemba, a popular member of parliament and owner of Moliere TV, was among people who spread scepticism of COVID-19 in the country. Honourable Lemba argued that COVID-19 was part of a political strategy to instil fear and panic in the public in order to facilitate plunder of the country's resources and attract foreign aid (Trapido & Inaka, 2020).

People in the DRC self-medicated with the various indigenous remedies recommended by migrants in the diaspora and not government-sanctioned measures. They drank and steamed with the concoctions cited earlier. A biochemist, Professor Théophile Mbemba, even advised people to take turmeric, ginger, garlic, onions, and *maniguette*, commonly known as "*Mondongo*" in Kinshasa and would say to them "consume eggplants because there are active ingredients, molecules, therefore antioxidants in its food products which are potential inhibitors of the COVID-19 protease" (Africanews, 2020).

Government responses

Following public outcry, Professor Muyembe retracted the statement he'd made earlier that the DRC would participate in COVID-19 vaccine trials. He did this on his official Facebook page in a video message where he said, "We are not going to start vaccination in the DRC without it being first tested in America and elsewhere. [. . .] I myself am Congolese and the Congolese will never be used as guinea pigs" (Ouest-France, 2020; DRC COVID-19 NEWS_Officiel, 2020). The government also authorised the use of hydroxychloroquine, azithromycin, and zinc as part of the protocol for treating COVID-19. Dr Raoult's and Dr Jerome Munyangi's messages seem to have helped influence the government in arriving at this position. The government of DRC encouraged the development of homemade remedies, like the Mana-COVID Antiviral (Actuality.CD, 2021). In his letter to the inventor, Congolese Phamacist Batangu, the Minister of Public Health Mr Eteni Longondo states that:

> Indeed, while welcoming the efforts made by your Research Center in response to the appeal launched by His Excellency the President of the Republic, Head of State for the daughters and sons of our country to find local therapy against the COVID-19 pandemic, I note, with satisfaction, the results obtained from clinical trials carried out in one of our hospitals. These clinical trial results being

conclusive and significant according to the investigator's report, the Minister of Health, through the Directorate of Pharmacy and Medicines, will support you for the rest of the process so that people sick with COVID-19 can find in this medicine an effective and safe remedy.

(Actualité.CD, 2021)

President Tshisekedi too made a visit to COVID-19 quarantine centres and medical facilities (Radio Okapi, 2020) in a bid to show that the government was concerned about people who were admitted to those institutions. During the visit, he promised that conditions in government-run health centres and facilities would be improved (Radio Okapi, 2020). The government also started giving regular updates on the pandemic and established COVID-19 testing centres in various hot-spot provinces like Haut Katanga, North Kivu, and South Kivu to speed up testing. More quarantine sites were also established in these provinces even though conditions were still alarming in some cases. The government also put up hand sanitising facilities and COVID-19 prevention messages in public places.

Congolese migrants and people back home

The Congolese migrants seem to have contributed to the creation of mistrust between ordinary people and the authorities responsible for public health in the DRC in the COVID-19 moment through health transnationalism. About 68% of the Congolese population is said to have developed misgivings about the reality and severity of COVID-19 (Target Sarl, 2020). The migrants also seemed to have been concerned with the prospect of people back home being treated as ignorant guinea pigs on which Western countries tested their vaccines. The migrants established strong bonds of trust with people in communities back home through health transnationalism. They gave COVID-19 information to people back home via social media that apparently influenced the behaviour of people and the authorities in the DRC. The migrants recommended indigenous remedies for COVID-19. The health transnationalism seemed so effective that the government rescinded its decision to run vaccine trials in the country. Social medias thus proved to be an effective tool for health transnationalism. It influenced public health officials and influenced ordinary people to demand acceptable responses from government. The government was forced to abandon plans to participate in vaccine trials.

Conclusion

Congolese migrants helped shape public perceptions and attitudes towards COVID-19 through the messages they shared with people back home via social media. They contributed to the spread of scepticism about the reality and existence of the disease in the DRC. Because of this, the majority of the people were reluctant to follow state-established measures and regulations to control the disease such as curfews. There was mistrust between the government, migrants, and ordinary people because of the messages that influenced public behaviour. Health transnationalism contributed to public resistance against COVID-19 vaccine trials in the DRC, which saw the government withdraw following pressure and tension on the streets and social media. Finally, people resorted to using local remedies like *kongo-bololo* and Manna-COVID as alternatives to those prescribed and sanctioned by the government and WHO. The government even got to a point where it recommended the use of hydroxychloroquine, azithromycin, and zinc as well as herbs as part of the protocol for treating COVID-19.

Notes

1 "We are not the pigs for COVID-19 vaccine trials" in French.
2 A very sour and bitter Congolese herb usually used in different indigenous medicine mixtures.
3 "Nous avons été choisis pour faire ces essais. Le vaccin sera produit soit aux États-Unis, soit au Canada, soit en Chine. Nous, nous sommes candidats pour faire les essais ici chez nous, a déclaré le professeur Muyembe. Peut-être vers le mois de juillet, août nous pourrons commencer déjà à avoir des essais cliniques de ce vaccin" (Ouest-France, April 2020). Authors' interpretation.
4 "Chers médecins, scientifiques et empires pharmaceutiques. Lorsque vous avez fini de tester vos vaccins Covid19 sur des animaux, avant même d'envisager de venir l'essayer sur des Africains, un peuple pour lequel vous n'avez jamais montré de considération, essayez sur vous-même" (Ouest-France, April 2020). Authors' interpretation.
5 Lingala for white skin.

References

Actualité, C. D. 2021. *RDC-COVID-19: Le ministre de la santé promet d'accompagner le pharmacien congolais géniteur du produit Manacovid lancé sur le marché*, Lundi 11 Janvier 2021–12:20. https://actualite.cd/2021/01/11/rdc-covid-19-le-ministre-de-la-sante-promet-daccompagner-le-pharmacien-congolais (accessed 3 February 2021).

Africanews. 2020. *DRC Uses Traditional Medicine in Virus Fight by Claudia Nsono.* www.africanews.com/2020/04/23/drc-uses-traditional-medicine-in-virus-fight// (accessed 21 August 2020).

Barraud, Y. 2020. *Didier Raoult dénonce la corruption, le Remdesivir et Gilead*, 17 November 2020. www.youtube.com/watch?v=TqiPK4pts7Y (accessed 19 December 2020).

Bauböck, R. 2003. Towards a political theory of migrant transnationalism. *International Migration Review*, 37(3): 700–723.

Bauböck, R. 2006. Citizenship and migration – Concepts and controversies. In *Migration and Citizenship: Legal Status, Rights and Political Participation*, edited by R. Bauböck, p. 128. Amsterdam: Amsterdam University Press.

Bauböck, R. and Faist, T. (eds.). 2010. *Diaspora and Transnationalism: Concepts, Theories and Methods*. Amsterdam: Amsterdam University Press.

BBC News. 2019. *Congo Student: 'I Skip Meals to Buy Online Data' by Gaius Kowene BBC News*, Kinshasa Published 24 November. www.bbc.com/news/world-africa-50516888 (accessed 20 August 2020).

BBC News. 2020. *Madagascar President's Herbal Tonic Fails to Halt COVID-19 Spike by Raïssa Ioussouf*, Antananarivo, Published 13 August. www.bbc.com/news/world-africa-53756752 (accessed 20 August 2020).

CGTN. 2020. *Tanzanian President Calls for Probe after Non-Human Samples Test Positive for COVID-19.* www.youtube.com/watch?v=6DjpTeTxD-0 (accessed 15 June 2020).

Coggon, J., Syrett, K. and Viens, A. M. 2017. *Public Health Law: Ethics, Governance, and Regulation.* London: Routledge.

Dawson, A. (ed.). 2011. *Public Health Ethics: Key Concepts and Issues in Policy and Practice.* Cambridge: Cambridge University Press.

Dawson, A. and Verweij, M. 2015. Public health: Beyond the role of the state. *Public Health Ethics,* 8(1): 1–3. https://doi.org/10.1093/phe/phv002

DRC COVID-19 NEWS_Officiel. 2020. *Essai Clinique d'un vaccin contre le Coronavirus en RDC: Muyembe calme le jeu !* 04 April. https://www.youtube.com/watch?v=y3aYnOB5azw (accessed 20 December 2020).

Flahaux, M. L. and De Haas, H. 2016. African migration: Trends, patterns, drivers. *Comparative Migration Studies,* 4(1). https://doi-org.uplib.idm.oclc.org/10.1186/s40878-015-0015-6

GSMA Intelligence. 2019. *Digital 2019 Democratic Republic of the Congo,* January (v01). www.slideshare.net/DataReportal/digital-2019-democratic- republic-of-the-congo-january-2019-v01 (accessed 8 December 2020).

Infobascongo.net. 2020. *Le Conseil des ministres présidé par Felix Tshisekedi critique la communication du ministre de la Santé sur le coronavirus.* By redaction 14 March. www.infobascongo.net/beta/2020/03/14/le-conseil-des-ministres-preside-par-felix-tshisekedi-critique-la-communication-du-ministre-de-la-sante-sur-le-coronavirus/ (accessed June 2020).

International Organisation of Migration (IOM). 2019. *World Migration Report 2020.* publications.iom.int/system/files/pdf/wmr_2020.pdf (accessed 10 December 2020).

Kennedy, J. 2020. Vaccine hesitancy: A growing concern. *Pediatric Drugs,* 22(2): 105–111.

Kirwin, M. and Anderson, J. 2018. Identifying the factors driving West African migration. In *West African Papers, No. 17.* Paris: OECD Publishing.

Kisangani, E. F. 2012. *Civil Wars in the Democratic Republic of Congo, 1960–2010.* Boulder: Lynne Rienner.

Lima, A. 2010. *Transnationalism: A New Mode of Immigrant Integration.* Boston: University of Massachusetts.

Marius Muhunga TV. 2020. *Interview Exclusive avec Dr Jerome Munyangi,* 25 April. www.youtube.com/watch?v=kgkIfiGILGU (accessed 20 August 2020).

Montague, D. 2002. Stolen goods: Coltan and conflict in the democratic republic of congo. *Sais Review,* 22(1): 103–118.

Mulongo, F. 2018. La Suisse et la diaspora Congolese: Résistants-PatriotesCombattants! *12 Mai 2018 Blog: Reveil Fm International by Freddy Mulongo.* https://blogs.mediapart.fr/freddy-mulongo/blog/120518/la-suisse-et-la-diaspora-congolaise-resistants-patriotes-combattants (accessed 4 April 2019).

Munthe, C. 2008. The goals of public health: An integrated, multidimensional model. *Public Health Ethics,* 1(1): 39–52.

Njoya, W. 2009. Lark mirror: African culture, masculinity, and migration to France in Alain Mabanckou's Bleu Blanc Rouge. *Comparative Literature Studies,* 46(2): 338–359.

Ouest-France. 2020. Coronavirus. La RDC candidate pour accueillir des essais d'un futur vaccin contre le COVID-19. *Agence France Press,* 3 April 2020. www.ouest-france.fr/sante/virus/coronavirus/coronavirus-la-rdc-candidate-pour-accueillir-des-essais-d-un-futur-vaccin-contre-le-covid-19-6799860 (accessed 22 August 2020).

Østergaard-Nielsen, E. (ed.). 2003. *International Migration and Sending Countries: Perceptions, Policies and Transnational Relations.* Basingstoke: Palgrave Macmillan.

Perullo, A. 2008. Rumba in the city of peace: Migration and the cultural commodity of Congolese music in dar es salaam, 1968–1985. *Ethnomusicology*, 52(2): 296–323.

Pötzschke, S. 2012. Measuring transnational behaviours and identities. https://www.ssoar.info/ssoar/handle/document/39532, (accessed 5 October 2020).

Radio Okapi. 2020. *Kinshasa: Félix Tshisekedi visite les hôpitaux désignés pour recevoir les malades de COVID-19*. https://www.radiookapi.net/2020/05/07/actualite/sante/kinshasa-felix-tshisekedi-visite-les-hopitaux-designes-pour-recevoir-les (accessed 5 June 2021).

Reliefweb. 2020a. *OCHA: République Démocratique du Congo: Carte des Zones de santé*, Juillet. https://reliefweb.int/map/democratic-republic-congo/r-publique-d-mocratique-du-congo-carte-des-zones-de-sant-juillet-2020 (accessed September 2020).

Reliefweb. 2020b. *Mobilisation against COVID-19 Draws on Ebola Response Experience*. https://reliefweb.int/report/democratic-republic-congo/mobilisation-against-covid-19-draws-ebola-response-experience (accessed 23 March 2021).

Reuters. 2020a. *We Are Not Guinea Pigs,' Say South African Anti-Vaccine Protesters*, July. www.youtube.com/watch?v=09PASKB3sgU (accessed 22 August 2020).

Reuters. 2020b. *Fact Check: RFID Microchips Will Not be Injected with the COVID-19 Vaccine, Altered Video features Bill and Melinda Gates and Jack Ma*, December. www.reuters.com/article/uk-factcheck-vaccine-microchip-gates-ma-idUSKBN28E286 (accessed January 2021).

Ryff, C. D. and Singer, B. 1998. The contours of positive human health. *Psychological Inquiry*, 9(1): 1–28.

SADC. 1999. *Protocol on Health in the Southern African Development Communities*. www.sadc.int/files/7413/5292/8365/Protocol_on_Health1999.pdf (accessed 19 December 2020).

Schiller, N. G., Basch, L. and Blanc-Szanton, C. 1992. Towards a definition of transnationalism. *Annals of the New York Academy of Sciences*, 645(1): iv–xiv.

Smith, B. J., Tang, K. C. and Nutbeam, D. 2006. WHO health promotion glossary: new terms. *Health Promotion International*, 21(4): 340–345.

Stasse, S., Vita, D., Kimfuta, J., Da Silveira, V. C., Bossyns, P. and Criel, B. 2015. Improving financial access to health care in the Kisantu district in the Democratic Republic of Congo: acting upon complexity. *Global Health Action*, 8(1): 25480.

Target Sarl. 2015. *Les Habitudes des Internautes (Aout 2015)*. www.target-sarl.cd/fr/content/rdc-84-des-congolais-accedent-internet-sur-support-mobile-selon-une-etude-de-target (accessed 23 December 2020).

Target Sarl. 2020. *Selon une enquête Target, 68% des Congolais ne croient toujours pas à la gravité de la COVID-19 by Target Research and Consulting*. www.target-sarl.cd/fr/content/selon-une-enquete-target-68-des-congolais-ne-croient-toujours-pas-la-gravite-de-la-covid-19 (accessed 23 December 2020).

Tedeschi, M., Vorobeva, E. and Jauhiainen, J. S. 2020. Transnationalism: Current debates and new perspectives. *GeoJournal*: 1–17.

Terrier, M. 2020. En RDC, les médecins déplorent la difficile gestion de la crise sanitaire. *LaCroix*, 18 June. www.la-croix.com/Monde/Afrique/En-RDC-medecins-deplorent-difficile-gestion-crise-sanitaire-2020-06–18–1201100478 (accessed December 2020).

Trapido, J. and Inaka, S. J. 2020. Kinshasa prepares for the pandemic to hit. *The Jacobin*. https://jacobinmag.com/2020/04/kinshasa-drc-democratic-republic-congo-covid-coronavirus/ (accessed 22 August 2020).

Tshimpaka, L. M. 2020. Intercontinental citizenship: Europe-based congolese migrants and their influence on homeland governance during 2011 DRC electoral crisis. *Migration Conundrums, Regional Integration and Development*: 117–162.

Tshimpaka, L. M. 2021. Solidarité en mouvement against homeland authoritarianism: Political transnationalism of Europe-based central African migrants. *Expanding Boundaries: Borders, Mobilities and the Future of Europe-Africa Relations*: 118–135.

Versteeg, M., Horley, T., Meng, A., Guim, M. and Guirguis, M. 2019. The law and politics of presidential term limit evasion. *Columbia Law Review, 2020; Virginia Public Law and Legal Theory Research Paper No. 2019–14.*

Vertovec, S. 2003. Migration and other modes of transnationalism: Towards conceptual cross-fertilization. *International Migration Review*, 37(3): 641–665.

Vertovec, S. 2009. *Transnationalism: Key Ideas*. London: Routledge.

Verweij, M. and Dawson, A. 2007. The meaning of 'public' in 'public health'. *Ethics, Prevention, and Public Health*: 13–29.

World Bank. 2020. *Interview with Professor Muyembe, the Ebola and COVID-19 Response Coordinator in the DRC: "Community Engagement and Awareness-Raising Campaigns Are Key to Winning the Battle"*. www.worldbank.org/en/news/feature/2020/05/19/interview-with-professor-muyembe-the-ebola-and-covid-19-response-coordinator-in-the-drc-community-engagement-and-awareness-raising-campaigns-are-key-to-winning-the-battle (accessed 23 March 2021).

World Health Organization. 1948. *Definition of Health*. www.who.int/suggestions/faq/zh/index. html (accessed 12 December 2020).

World Health Organization. 2021. *Coronavirus Disease (COVID-19) Pandemic: Number at a Glance*. www.who.int/emergencies/diseases/novel-coronavirus-2019 (accessed 24 February 2021).

10

"#CORONA JIHAD"

Remanufacturing Islamophobic narratives during COVID-19 in contemporary India

Sayan Dey

In Medias Res: "#CoronaJihad"

From 13 March to 15 March 2020, a Tablighi Jamaat gathering was organised at Nizamuddin Markaz in Delhi. Tablighi Jamaat is an "Islamic reformist movement founded in 1927 whose followers travel across the world on proselytizing missions" (Desai & Amarasingam, 2020: 34). On 16 March 2020, the chief minister of New Delhi announced that "no religious, social, political gatherings of more than 50 people are allowed in Delhi till March 31" (Haider, 2020: 4). In spite of this official announcement, it was found that the Jamaat attendees continued to stay close to each other and gather at the Markaz. The Tablighi Jamaat, which saw a gathering of "more than 4500 people from the world over" (Trivedi, 2020: 7), has been identified as India's "largest COVID-19 cluster" (Trivedi, 2020: 6) to date. Undoubtedly, such a gathering during a disease outbreak is a highly condemnable act, but the way it was communally and racially condemned by the individuals and the media was highly problematic in many ways. Immediately after this incident, groups of Hindu fanatics, who were already manufacturing and propagating Islamophobic narratives since the pre-COVID times, received further impetus from various governing institutions and the media to justify why the Muslims should be driven out of India and why India should be developed into a Hindu-dominated nation. In order to logically systematise these narratives, the gathering at the Markaz was identified by several political organisations, media houses, and individuals on social media as a deliberate *Jihadic* exercise to spread coronavirus in India. For instance, within a few days of the Jamaat gathering, an individual posted a picture on Twitter, which identified the Muslims as *coronavirus* in India. The picture made an effort to show that prior to COVID-19, the Muslims tried to spread violence through bombs, and during COVID-19, they have been spreading violence through coronavirus. Another caricature, which was

DOI: 10.4324/9781003415121-10

posted in one of the leading English-language newspapers in India called *The Hindu* on 26 March 2020, portrayed the coronavirus as a terrorist in Muslim attire, who is pointing a gun towards the planet Earth.

The Karnataka BJP (Bharatiya Janata Party) MP (Member of Parliament) Shobha Karandlaje observed: "Most of the attendees of the event are untraceable. There seems to be 'corona Jihadi plan' behind that meeting" (cited in Ghosh, 2020: 11). These instances reveal that by (mis)interpreting the Tablighi Jamaat gathering as a deliberate attempt to spread coronavirus amongst the Indians (especially the non-Muslim Indians) by the Muslims, India seems to uphold the epistemic racial ideologies of a Westernised, modern, colonial, and capitalist world system (Grosfoguel, 2008: 36). This socially, culturally, racially, communally, and politically toxic world system consistently creates "institutions and structures of power that sustains colonizer-colonized relations of exploitation, domination and repression" (Ndlovu-Gatsheni, 2020: 2). The institutions and structures of power "[invade] the mental universe of the people" (Ndlovu-Gatsheni, 2020: 5), destabilise them, and then "[commit] 'crimes' such as *epistemicide* (where you kill and displace pre-existing knowledges), *linguicide* (killing and displacing the languages of a people and imposing your own) and *culturecide* (where you kill or replace the cultures of a people)" (Ndlovu-Gatsheni, 2020: 6). In an identical manner, the different institutions and structures of power, as manufactured and preserved by the media houses and different socio-political organisations in contemporary India, have been committing various forms of epistemicides, linguicides, and culturecides against the Muslims. The Islamophobic narratives have given birth to corona-logy. "Corona-logy can be defined as a neo-colonial and a neo-racial civilizational project that uses the logic of a disease named COVID-19 to unpack newly configured social groups, who are being microscopically confined within the narrow chambers of racialization, criminalization, victimization and dehumanization" (Dey, 2020: 51). This civilisation project not only enables the gatekeepers of the institutions and the structures of power to unburden themselves from all forms of humanitarian responsibilities but also allows them to hide their "sinister motives" (Ndlovu-Gatsheni, 2020: p. 7) successfully. Shweta Desai and Amarnath Amarasingam argue that during COVID-19 the hidden sinister motives of the Hindu fanatics have reconfigured the practice of Islamophobia in India through analysing the Muslims as "1) contaminated/contaminating 2) as uncivilized 3) as deceptive, and 4) as anti-national jihadists or terrorists" (2020: 41). This process of reconfiguration is not a sudden act, but a thoroughly researched and a well-outlined infodemic[1] project, which is firmly supported by tools like verbal rumours, fake videos, false news reports, communal propagandas, etc.

On 12 May 2020, in the Telinipara region of Hooghly district, a Hindu mob attacked the house of 20-year-old Hena Tabassum and burnt it down to ashes. According to Hena Tabassum: "We were fasting for Ramadan. It was around 12:30 p.m. Suddenly the mob attacked. They threw bombs, petrol bombs, and also dropped a gas cylinder into the room, before setting it aflame. I was inside the room. I was rescued by some neighbors before I got burned. Everything in the room turned to ashes" (cited in Rahman, 2020: 3). Police investigations revealed that the mob violence was triggered by a rumour that "hundreds of Muslims had been infected with COVID-19 and were infecting members of the town's Hindu majority" (Rahman, 2020: 6). On 23 April 2020, an imam from the Humnabad region of Karnataka named Hafiz Mohammed Naseerudin was assaulted by a police officer for being a Muslim. As Naseerudin shared: "I am an Imam, so I look and dress very Muslim. I also have a long beard. The cop started hitting me and saying that it is because of me and my community that this disease is spreading" (Regan, Sur and Sud, 2020: 11). On 2 April 2020 a fake video was published against the Muslims, which showed that men from the Dawoodi Bohra[2] community are licking utensils and "deliberately spreading Coronavirus in the country amidst the COVID-19 pandemic" (Chattopadhyay, 2020: 14). A thorough fact-checking revealed that before being washed the Dawoodi Bohra community members were licking the utensils because according to their traditional practice they cannot waste a single amount of food. Therefore, prior to washing the utensils, they were licking them as clean as possible. On 3 April 2020 a Muslim man named Sheru was arrested in the Raisen district of Madhya Pradesh under sections "269, 270 of the Indian penal code. Section 269 of the IPC deals with negligent act that is likely to spread infection of disease dangerous to life and section 270 deals with malignant act, which is likely to spread infection of disease dangerous to life" (Explained Desk, 2020: 12). The arrest was made on the basis of the video, which showed that a Muslim fruit-seller was spitting on the fruits that he was selling. Several social media users claimed that through spitting, the man is deliberately trying to spread coronavirus. Though the content of the video is true, it was found that the recording dates back to 12 February 2020 and has no connection with the intention of spreading COVID-19. His daughter also revealed that Sheru was unconsciously spitting on the fruits because he is mentally imbalanced and has been battling with psychological diseases for the past few years.

This culture of communal scapegoating during pandemics is not new. Asim Ali, a researcher at the Center for Policy Research in New Delhi, observes: "Pandemics have a long history of scapegoating, starting from the Bubonic Plague in the 14th century, where Jews were accused of poisoning wells and spreading the contagion. . . . During times of crisis people revert to their identities and search for others to blame for their problems" (cited in Krishnan, 2020: 13). The continuous exercise of scapegoating certain communities during pandemics generates, normalises, and systematises a continuous pattern of blaming that permanently dehumanises the social, cultural, political, racial, and economic existence of a particular community. The Muslims in India have been undergoing a similar experience during COVID-19. Vidya Krishnan, a senior health journalist, argues:

You cannot isolate the February riots in Delhi from what happened through much of April in everyday media briefings where the Health Ministry and Home Ministry were actively painting a target on the backs of one community. . . .

This is a continuing pattern of blaming those who get infected instead of taking human and scientific remedial measures like affordable healthcare, better contact tracing and putting data in the public domain.

(cited in Vetticad, 2020: 10)

These patterns of blaming, as put forth by the individuals, media houses, and the socio–political institutions develop, multiple *narratives of distractions*, which effectively masquerade the realities, on the one side, and manipulate falsehoods as realities, on the other. This is why the Tablighi Jamaat gathering has been solely held responsible for the alarming rise in COVID-19 infections in India during the months of March, April, and May, while the issue of various Hindu-centric social, cultural, political, and religious gatherings has been strategically and systemically ignored by the individuals and the media houses. Niharika Sharma, a social media reporter, in one of her articles notes the following non-Islamic socio-cultural gatherings that took place before, during, and after the Tablighi Jamaat congregation:

a. Rashtrapati Bhawan, New Delhi: On 8 March 2020 as a part of the International Women's Day an award ceremony was organized at the Rashtrapati Bhawan (presidential palace) and it was attended by a large number of people across the country. It is important to note that the event was organised during the time when the rise of COVID-19 cases was already confirmed in New Delhi.
b. Aatukal Pongala, Thiruvananthapuram: A ten-day Hindu religious festival called Aatukal Pongala was organised in the city of Thiruvananthapuram, Kerala and it started on the same day of the award ceremony at Rashtrapati Bhawan. The festival was organised with the prior permission of the state government of Kerala. When the government was interrogated, it justified the commencement of this festival by saying that as everything was already planned out, therefore, in spite of the COVID-19 outbreak, they gave permission for the celebration of Aatukal Pongala festival. On the second day of the festival, Kerala had already recorded 43 COVID-19 cases.
c. Ram Navami, Ayodhya: A three-week nationwide lockdown was announced by the prime minister of India on 24 March 2020. But the chief minister of Uttar Pradesh, Yogi Adityanath, defied the very first day of the lockdown by organising and attending a public event in Ayodhya on the Hindu religious occasion of Ram Navami.[3]
d. Wedding in Karnataka: On 15 March 2020 the state government of Karnataka imposed a state-wide ban on any form of public gatherings due to the COVID-19 outbreak. On the same day of the imposition of the state-wide ban several hundred guests attended the wedding of state legislator Mahantesh Kavatgimath's daughter. In fact, the wedding gathering was also attended by the chief minister of Karnataka.
e. Sikh fair in Punjab: From 10–12 March 2020 a Sikh fair was organised in Punjab, and it was attended by a coronavirus-infected 70-year-old Sikh man. Later on, the man died due to COVID-19, and he came in contact with almost 40,000 people.

These examples not only reveal the collective hatred against the Muslims during COVID-19 in particular but also unpacks how Islamophobia, in general, creates "an exaggerated fear, hatred, and hostility toward Islam and Muslims that is perpetuated by negative stereotypes resulting in bias, discrimination, and the marginalization and exclusion of Muslims from social, political and civic life" (Ali et al., 2011: 9).

With respect to these arguments, the chapter has been divided into four sections. The introductory section titled "*In Medias Res*: '#CoronaJihad'" sets the thematic and the theoretical tone of this chapter through various ethnographic narratives. The term *Corona Jihad* was first used on Twitter by a Hindu man who accused the Muslims of practising Jihad through spreading coronavirus. This section discusses the various social and cultural factors that provoked the development of such anti-Muslim attitudes and normalised the Muslims as *Corona Jihadis* during the COVID-19 pandemic. The section also discusses its impact on the Muslim community in India.

The second section titled "Hindu-centric Islamophobia: A Socio-Historical Overview of Anti-Muslim Politics in Contemporary India" positions the problem of anti-Muslim practices during COVID-19 in India within the wider epistemological and ontological frameworks of Islamophobia as preserved and practised through anti-Muslim sentiments in contemporary India. The section not only elaborates on the various socio-historical factors that motivate the practice of anti-Muslim politics in contemporary India but also outlines how the phenomenon of Islamophobia, apart from unleashing physical violence against the Muslims, unleashes epistemic and ontological violence as well. The third section titled "Resistance: The RDC (Realisation-Depolarisation-Collaboration) Model" discusses the possible initiatives that are currently being taken and that can be taken in the future to resist the rising practices of Islamophobia in contemporary India. The final section, "Conclusion", summarises the various arguments and findings of this chapter.

Hindu-centric Islamophobia: a socio-historical overview of anti-Muslim politics in contemporary India

In the article "A Measure of Islamophobia" (2014) Salman Sayyid philosophises:

> Islamophobia is a concept that emerges precisely to do the work that categories like racism were not doing. It names something that needs to be named. Its continual circulation in public debate testifies to ways in which it hints at something that needs to be addressed. What it names, of course, remains a matter of dispute.
> *(p. 21)*

The culture of categorising and naming Islamophobic practices in India is not new, and the country has experienced various forms of racially, communally, religiously, and politically focused Hindu-centred anti-Muslim violence in the past.

Kolkata riots in 1964

In the year 1964 riots broke out between the Hindus and Muslims in Kolkata, and more than 100 people were killed and 400 people were injured. The riot was motivated by the "arson attacks and looting against Muslims. . . . Most of the riots have resulted in the looting and burning of Muslim property" (BBC News, 2020: 16).

Gujarat riots of 1969

On 18 September 1969 thousands of Muslim men and women gathered for Urs[4] near a Jagannatha Temple.[5] Apart from the Muslim gathering, several Hindu monks also gathered near the temple. As one of the monks was adjusting his robes, his stick accidently hit one of the Muslim women who was standing with her daughter in the queue near the *dargah*. Due this incident a verbal spat broke out between the Hindus and Muslims which ultimately culminated into physical clashes. The Muslim men chased the monks inside the temple and injured them with sticks and stones. As an act of retaliation, large numbers of Muslims were attacked and their houses and shops were ransacked on 19 September 1969. The pattern of the violence reveals that it was well planned and was clearly underlined with anti-Muslim intentions. Saquib Salim in his article titled "Gujarat Riots – 1969" (2020) notes:

> The mob showed a calculated sense of discrimination. Muslim shops in Hindu-owned buildings were plundered but not set on fire; similar shops in Muslim-owned buildings were set on fire; shops run by a Hindu and Muslim in partnership remained undisturbed. . . . No fire-brigades came to the help of the Muslim shopkeepers most of whom were themselves not on the site.
>
> *(p. 18)*

Several trains were also burnt and Muslim passengers were attacked, raped, and killed. The mobs were let loose, and the state government hardly played any role to bring the riots under control.

Moradabad riots in 1980

On 13 August 2020, as the Muslims gathered outside the Moradabad Mosque to offer prayers on the occasion of Eid, the police and the provincial armed constabulary opened fire on the devotees. It was reported that around 40,000 Muslims gathered and more than 300 were killed. In the book *Riot After Riot* (1988) M.J. Akbar says:

> Men of the Provincial Armed Constabulary opened fire on about 40,000 Muslims while they were at Eid prayers. No one knows exactly how many people died. What is known is that the incident at Moradabad was not a Hindu-Muslim riot but a calculated cold-blooded massacre of Muslims by a rabidly communal police force which tried to cover up its genocide by making it out to be a Hindu-Muslim riot.
>
> *(p. 91)*

In the article titled "Remembering 1980 Moradabad Muslim Massacre" (2017), Sharjeel Imam and Saquib Salim have compared the Moradabad riots with the Jail-lanwala Bagh massacre, which took place on 13 April 1919. They said:

> Compare that to Jallianwala Bagh, where thousands had gathered on the day of Baisakhi to celebrate and protest. The army under the command of Dyer opened fire, killing around 400 people. The similarities do not end there. In both cases the victims were fired upon and confined to closed spaces with only one exit point which was blocked.
>
> *(p. 20)*

Nellie massacre in 1983

The Nellie massacre took place in Nellie and several other villages in Assam on the morning of 18 February 1983. The attack was planned and executed by the All Assam Students' Union (AASU), and it was directed against the Muslim "foreign-ers"[6]. The AASU did not want the inclusion of the Muslim "foreigners" in the state electoral process of Assam, and therefore the Muslims were massacred. In *The Nellie Massacre of 1983: Agency of Rioters* (2013), Makiko Kimura writes: "150,000 armed men in uniform were in place to ensure law and order – one army man for 57 vot-ers – turning Assam into a military background rather than a political state suitable democratically elect political representatives" (p. 112). On the day of the massacre, Hemendra Narayan, a journalist, reported: "In a systematic manner the houses of the Muslim settlements at Demalgaon . . . were burnt . . . the entire picturesque green hill range was covered with thick black could of smoke, which even the mid-day sun failed to penetrate. It was darkness at noon" (cited in Choudhary, 2019: 10).

Bhiwandi riots in 1984

Bhiwandi is a city in the Thane district of Maharashtra. Police investigations have re-vealed that this attack was collaboratively instigated by various Hindu fanatic groups of Maharashtra, like Shiv Sena, Patil Pawan, and Hindu Mahasabha, against the Mus-lim residents of Bhiwandi. Prior to the outbreak of the riots, during Maha Sangh's meeting at Chowpatty (a locality near Mumbai) on 21 April 1985, Bal Thackeray addressed the Muslims as *landiya*[7] and declared that "the Muslims are spreading like cancer and should be operated upon like cancer" (cited in Kapoor, 1984: 17). So, on 7 May 1985 when the riots broke out in Bhiwandi, the Muslims were targeted and killed by the Hindu fanatics.

Hashimpura massacre in 1987

On the night of 22 May 1987 42 young Muslim men were picked up by paramilitary soldiers from their houses in Hashimpura, which is located near the city of Meerut in the state of Uttar Pradesh. After being picked up, the men were taken to the banks of the Hindon Canal, where they were shot from behind and then their bullet-ridden bodies were thrown into the canal. According to Harsh Mander:

> The men were guilty of no crime, and were chosen for slaughter by the paramilitary soldiers only because of the god they worshipped and their youth. Not a single person has been punished for this crime despite heroic and dogged battles for justice for three decades by the indigent survivors of the slain men.
>
> *(2017: 14)*

Muzaffarpur riots in 2013

The city of Muzaffarpur is located in the state of Bihar and on 7 September 2013 riots broke out between the Hindus and the Muslims. Centrally, the riots targeted the Muslim residents of Muzaffarpur, and it was driven by a fake video clip, which showed that two Hindu boys are being beaten by a Muslim mob. Later on, the police investigations revealed that the video clip was fake and it was shot in Pakistan in 2011. During the violence the Muslim homes, shops, and mosques were exclusively targeted and burnt down. A news article by BBC on 25 September 2013 revealed that "the violence that followed left dozens more dead and forced 40,000 mainly Muslims, to flee their homes. More than 18,000 people still remain in the camps" (p. 23).

Apart from generating physical violence against the Muslims in India, the collaborative efforts of the individuals, media houses, and states have led to the development of epistemological and ontological Islamophobia as well. The epistemological and ontological Islamophobia that is practised today in India is highly identical to the anti-Islamic ideologies that were once socio-politically implemented by the British colonisers in India as a part of their *divide and rule* framework (Singh, 2017: 2; Pillalamarri, 2019: 4; Matharu, 2019: 5). As a part of their divide and rule framework, the British argued that "Islam was incompatible with science and philosophy" (Ernst, 2003: 112). Through systemically, epistemically, and ontologically denying the social, cultural, historical, and philosophical existence of the Muslims, India is following a similar framework. In order to deliberately disown, dehumanise, and permanently erase the socio-historical contributions of the Muslims towards the development of Indian society and culture, the Islamic names of railway stations, cities, and villages are being removed and are being rechristened with Hindu names.

For example, the name of the railway station in Mughal Sarai, which is located in the Chandauli district of Uttar Pradesh, was changed from Mughal Sarai to Pandit Deendayal Upadhyaya. Earlier the station was named Mughal Sarai because the city of Mughal Sarai was found and laid by the Mughals. But in 2017, under the rule of the right-wing Bharatiya Janta Party (BJP) government the station was renamed after Pandit Deendayal Updhayaya, who was a right-wing Indian politician and an active member of BJP. In 2018, the city of Allahabad in Uttar Pradesh was renamed Prayagraj. Originally, the city was built in 1583 by Mughal Emperor Akbar and it was named Allahabad, which means *City of God*. The state government justified this act of rechristening by saying that the name Prayagraj will restore the "city's ancient identity as a major Hindu pilgrimage centre" (Biswas, 2018: 17). In the same year, three villages in Rajasthan, namely Ismail Khurd, Miyonka Bara, and Narpada, were "renamed as Pichanwa Khurd, Mahesh Nagar and Narpura respectively" (PTI, 2018: 18). Gaganpreet Singh from Delhi University believes that these acts are "rooted in the nationalisation of heritage" (cited in Biswas, 2018: 12). This systematic process of disempowering India's Muslims and denying them "a stake in the country's history" (Biswas, 2018: 17) is also being practised through the Citizenship Amendment Bill (CAB), which was passed in 2019. Meenakshi Ganguly, the South Asia director for Human Rights Watch, says: "The bill uses the language of refuge and sanctuary, but discriminates on religious grounds in violation of international law" (cited in Human Rights Watch, 2019: 21). Though the aim of the bill is to protect such people "who were forced or compelled to seek shelter in India due to persecution on the ground of religion" (ET Online, 2019: 16), the draft clearly favours the Hindus and other non-Muslim immigrants over the Muslims. This can be clearly understood through Home Minister Amit Shah's speech, which he delivered during an election rally in New Delhi in 2018. In his speech, he indirectly demonised the Muslims as infiltrators and terrorists by saying: "Illegal immigrants are like termites and they are eating the food that should go to our poor and they are taking our jobs. They carry out blasts in our country and so many of our people die" (cited in Human Rights Watch, 2019: 9).

The government's version of Hindu-centric Islamophobia seems to adopt Hitler's dictatorial model of anti-Semitic ideologies against the Muslims through building detention camps in Assam. Though the government of India has brushed away the news of detention camps as rumours, several news sources have categorically revealed that ten detention camps are being constructed in Assam for the illegal immigrants (also read as Muslims), and some of them have already started functioning (Banerji, 2019: 2; Hussain, 2020: 4; Pradhan, 2020: 7; Siddique, 2020: 8; Karmakar, 2020: 5) The detention camps, with boundary walls and watch towers, are trying to naturalise epistemological and ontological Islamophobia through a simultaneous process of criminalisation, victimisation, and discrimination of Muslims in general and Muslim immigrants in particular. Sigal Samuel observes:

> If you live in Assam and your name does not appear on the NRC, the burden of proof is on you to prove that you're a citizen. . . . You do get the chance to appeal to a Foreigner's Tribunal. If they don't buy your claim citizenship, you can appeal to the High Court of Assam or even the Supreme Court. But, if all that fails, you can be sent to one of the 10 mass detention camps the government plans to build, complete with boundary walls and watch towers. . . . Even nursing mothers and children will be held there.
>
> *(2019: 19)*

Shashi Tharoor identifies this process of systemic and epistemic erasure of Islamic existence in contemporary India as "a cynical political exercise to single out and disenfranchise an entire community in India and in doing so, a betrayal of all that was good and noble about our civilization" (cited in Human Rights Watch, 2019: 3).

These Hindu-centric anti-Islamic practices within and outside the parameters of communal violence during COVID-19 can be analysed further through focusing on the various social, cultural, political, and geographical dimensions of Islamophobia.

Brand Islamophobia

Islamophobia, especially after the election of the BJP government in 2014, has gained a brand value. Prior to and after the election of the BJP government in power, several politicians from the government have been found delivering anti-Muslim speeches and physically as well as ideologically provoking the Hindus to act against Muslims. On 3 April 2014, Amit Shah (the current home minister), during the pre-election rally, targeted his speech against the Muslims by saying: "This election is about voting out the government that protect and gives compensation to those who killed Jats[8]. It is about badla (revenge) and protecting izzat (honour)" (HT Correspondent, 2014: 14). This habitual hatred towards Muslims has been converted into a creative branding exercise through closing websites that voiced protest against Islamophobia; through arresting, imposing false criminal charges, and imprisoning individuals for protesting against Hindu fanaticism; through creating virtual *war rooms* and tracking media personnel and reporters who speak against the ruling government; through creating animated videos and justifying hatred against Muslims; and through opening websites that document hate and violence. In *Islamophobia in India: Stoking Bigotry* (2019), Paula Thompson, Rhonda Itaoui, and Hatem Bazian analyse how the social, cultural, political, and media branding of Islamophobia widely assisted the BJP government to come to power in 2014. According to them: "Polarizing politics are lucrative at the ballot box where individuals affiliated with stoking communal hate and violence are actually four times more likely to win than others" (pp. 58–60). In spite of implementing *polarisation politics* as a tool to discharge violence against Muslims, especially during COVID-19, brand Islamophobia has ideologically hypnotised several Hindu fanatics, who justify, celebrate, and acknowledge the anti-Muslim sentiments of the BJP government in a naturalised manner.

Geographical Islamophobia

Brand Islamophobia gained further value in India through its selective geographical spatialisation across the country. In other words, "Islamophobia is spatialized through communal violence, attacks and contestations over the rights for Muslim neighborhoods and places of worship to exist in the Indian national space" (Thompson et al., 2019: 62). So, the greatest amount of anti-Muslim communal violence can be usually seen in the states of Uttar Pradesh, Telangana, Haryana, Maharashtra, Rajasthan, Madhya Pradesh, Bihar, Jharkhand, Assam, and West Bengal. These acts of spatially induced Hindu-centric Islamophobic violence are deliberately instigated to deliver "nationalistic and exclusionary message[s] against non-Hindu minorities" (Thompson et al., 2019: 63).

The nationalistic and exclusionary messages are delivered through the vandalization of Muslim sites like mosques and monuments; through infiltrating the Muslim sites and spying on the Muslim communities; through preaching anti-Muslim propaganda in Muslim neighbourhoods; through creating ghettos in the form of detention centres; and through criminalising, racializing, and communalising Islamic religious gatherings and blacklisting Islamic religious places in the form of *lockdowns,* as happened in the case of the Tablighi Jamaat gathering at Nizamuddin Markaz. For instance, on 6 December 1992 the Babri Masjid (Babri Mosque) was illegally demolished by a group of activists from Vishwa Hindu Parishad[9] (VHP) and other Hindu-centric right-wing groups in Ayodhya, Uttar Pradesh. In order to justify their act, the VHP claimed that historically and mythically Ayodhya is the birthplace of Lord Rama; therefore, the mosque cannot exist there. On 31 May 2018 a group of men from the Newal village of Haryana invaded the mosque of the village, "beat up the people offering Namaz[10] and also destroyed the loud speakers. The young men also issued threats to the ones offering prayers" (Staff Reporter, 2018: 4). On 10 June 2018 a group of members from the VHP barged onto the campus of the Taj Mahal in Agra and pulled down a steel gate, which was installed for ticket collection from the visitors. In order to justify the act a VHP leader said: "The gate was blocking the way to a 400-year-old temple of Hindu god Shiva" (cited in Beaty, 2018: 11). But the Archaeological Survey of India (ASI) dismissed this claim by saying that there is an alternative way to reach the temple. During the communal riots in New Delhi in 2020, "a mosque and a dargah was vandalised before being set afire . . . in northeast Delhi" (Press Trust of India, 2020). Sajid Ibrahim, a resident from Chand Bagh of northeast Delhi, questioned: "Seeing the shrine in such a condition is very hurtful. Did any Hindu shrine get vandalised this way?" (cited in Press Trust of India, 2020: 8). These consistent practices of geographical Islamophobia continue to take place during COVID-19, and the communalisation and spatialisation of the Tablighi Jamaat gathering at Nizamuddin Markaz, which has already been discussed in the introductory section, is a glaring example.

Gastronomic Islamophobia

The government of India, in collaboration with the Ministry of Environment, imposed a ban on the sale and purchase of cattle for the purpose of slaughtering at animal markets across the country, under the Prevention of Cruelty to Animal Act on 26 May 2017. Though the ban was officially imposed on cattle slaughter in general, centrally, the target was to prevent the Muslims from consuming beef. The imposition of the ban not only systematically disrupted the habitual food and culinary practices of the Muslims but also heavily impacted their economic modes of existence. To elaborate further, the socio-economic existence of the Muslims whose mode of existence exclusively depended on slaughtering cows, selling beef, and/or cooking and serving beef dishes in the restaurants was completely dismantled.

In Rajasthan a Muslim truck driver, who was transporting cows to a village in Haryana for slaughtering and consumption, was killed on 4 April 2017. The other people in the truck were also injured, after a mob, "reportedly counting hundreds, intercepted the cattle truck on a highway, and dragged out and assaulted the Muslims who were trying to transport the cows to their home state of Haryana" (DW, 2017: 17). In New Delhi, a self-claimed animal rights activist group beat up three Muslim men "for transporting buffaloes" (Human Rights Watch, 2017) in a truck on 22 April 2017. The police, instead of arresting the assaulters, arrested the victims under a law that prevents cruelty against animals. Meenakshi Ganguly said: "Self-appointed cow protectors driven by irresponsible populism are killing people and terrorizing minority communities" (cited in Human Rights Watch, 2017: 1). A group of Muslim men were assaulted by a mob of 20 Hindu men in a train on 23 June 2017 for consuming beef. In fact, "one of the boys, 16-year-old Junaid Khan, was killed in the assault carried out by a mob of about 20 men" (BBC News, 2017: 11). James Bennet in his article "India's Cattle Trader Fear Ruin" (2017) argues that "the ban is an attempt to control what people eat [and] . . . for imposing Hindu values" (p. 4). In the state of Jharkhand, on 29 June 2017 a Muslim man named Alimuddin Ansari was pulled out from his car and beaten to death by a mob of Hindu men for transporting beef (Safi, 2018: 13). A Muslim man named Shaukat Ali was attacked by a group of Hindus in Assam for selling beef on 8 April 2019. He was not only physically assaulted but also was referred to as a Bangladeshi and was compelled to eat pork (Niazi, 2019: 12). On 31 July 2020 a Muslim man named Lukmaan in the Gurgaon district of Haryana was beaten by a mob of Hindu men for transporting buffalo meat in his truck (Dawn, 2020: 14). Investigations from the police have revealed that the Muslim man was attacked for two major reasons. Firstly, he was attacked for transporting buffalo meat. Secondly, he was attacked because they believed that the man was deliberately trying to spread the infection of COVID-19 through selling the meat.

These experiences of physical, epistemological, and ontological Islamophobia, as elaborated in this section, unfold the various social, cultural, political, communal, geographical, historical, gastronomic, and economic structures that are being implemented to justify the Islamophobic template of *Corona Jihad*, which has been strategically engineered by the Hindu fanatics against the Muslims through the weapon of coronalogy in contemporary India. The following section proposes a possible model to resist and decapitate Islamophobic practices in India during and after the pandemic of COVID-19.

Resistance: the RDC (realisation-depolarisation-collaboration) model

As discussed earlier, Islamophobia is not only a physical construct but also an "ideological construct" (Sheehi, 2011: 78; Bazian, 2018: 7). As a result, through a range of possible strategies, it is important to resist and disarm Islamophobia physically as well as ideologically, so that the habitual experiences of existence can be perceived in an independent and holistic manner. Aditya Nigam believes that this experience of independent and holistic existence is a "necessary preliminary step towards epistemic reconstitution" (2020: 52).

Some of the possible strategies that could be undertaken to epistemically reconstitute the habitual, social, cultural, political, religious, and economic existence of the Muslims in contemporary India and to build a non-Islamophobic society are as follows:

a. Realisation: Amongst several factors, two major factors that contribute towards physical and ideological Islamophobia is the lack of self-realisation and blind faith in rumours. This lack of self-realisation and blind faith in rumours distract individuals from investigating the original facts and draw them into someone else's propagandist constructs. Therefore, it is important to avoid these physical, ideological, epistemological, and ontological traps and engage in the practices of self-awareness and self-realisation. Instead of blindly believing and acting on the basis of the information as delivered by media houses and politicians against Muslims, it is important for the common people to make an effort to understand the issues and challenges as holistically and genuinely as possible. Police investigations reveal that a majority of Islamophobic attacks have been motivated by rumours. It can only be countered when individuals implement their own thought processes and understandings instead of relying on somebody else. For instance, if we again go back to the incident of the Tablighi Jamaat gathering at Nizamuddin Markaz, which sparked the phenomenon of Corona Jihad, and re-investigate, then the communal propaganda of the media and the central government of India behind the criminalisation of the event cannot be ignored. The communal propaganda emerged so successfully because most of the people did not bother to investigate and analyse the event from their respective viewpoints. This situation can be identified as a form of epistemic lethargy,[11] which has been strategically generated by several fake news platforms whose misleading information is easily available as compared to those whose information needs to be excavated through the process of self-investigation, self-awareness, and self-realisation. This process of resistance against habitual Islamophobia appears to be highly common and easily implementable, but, unfortunately, it has hardly been put into practice to date.

b. Depolarisation: The practices of self-investigation, self-awareness, and self-realisation also lead to the evolution of a set of social, cultural, communal, political, religious, and economic practices which Boaventura de Sousa Santos identifies as "depolarised pluralities" (2016: 106). He also adds that "there are three major dimensions of the construction of depolarised pluralities inside transformative collective actions: depolarisation through intensification of mutual communication and intelligibility; depolarisation through searching inclusive organizational forms; depolarisation through concentration on productive questions" (2016: 108). Through these practices of mutual communication, creating inclusive organisational forms and asking productive questions, there lies a possibility of countering Islamophobia in India during and after the pandemic of COVID-19. It is so because the adoption of such depolarised plural practices will enable individuals to disentangle themselves from the narrow contours of communal and political propagandism of the media houses and religion-based vote bank politics of the political parties, which India is experiencing currently. If a certain section of the Muslim community is found to defy the lockdown protocols and to risk the lives of civilians through conducting socio-religious gatherings in the name of Islam during COVID-19, then the solution is not to generate Islamophobia and create communal cleavages by denigrating their religious beliefs and socio-cultural practices. Instead, it is important to interact with them, to identify the root causes behind such ignorance, and to create health and medical awareness amongst them in a rational and inclusive manner. This practice of interaction should not only be applied in a definite situational context (like COVID-19) but should also be adopted as a cultural habit in the coming days.

c. Collaboration: The rationality and inclusivity can only be successfully nurtured through generating collaborative socio-cultural and religious practices between Muslims and non-Muslims. Specifically, with respect to Hindu-Muslim harmony, several socio-religious collaborations have taken place since the pre-European colonial era in India. The third Mughal emperor Akbar offered grants to Hindu temples and temple-servants for constructing around 35 temples in Vrindavan, Mathura, and other adjacent areas (Dogra, 2019). His son Jahangir "continued the tradition of supporting a multi-faith India by making significant additions to the grants approved by his father. He added at least two temples to the list" (Tasci, 2020: 15). Historical records reveal that during the emperorship of Jahangir around "30 hectares of land" were given to five families of temple caretakers (Dogra, 2016: 8). In case of any issue, the Hindu priests approached Jahangir and senior officials for assistance.

This tradition of Hindu-Muslim collaborations also continues in the contemporary era. In North Guwahati of Assam, for centuries, a Muslim family has been taking care of a Shiva temple.[12] A 73-year-old man named Haji Matibar Rahman, who currently takes care of the temple, says: "Apart from the Hindus, lots of Muslims also come here and offer 'dua' (prayers). They have a lot of faith as prayers get answered. The number of devotees coming here over the years has only increased" (cited in IANS, 2019: 12). For the last 26 years, a Muslim community in the city of Muzaffarnagar in Bihar has been taking care of an abandoned Hindu temple. Mohd Dilshad observes: "Twenty-six years later, this shrine is still maintained by its Muslim neighbours, who clean it daily, whitewash it every Diwali and protect it from squatters and stray animals" (2018: 4).

During the month of Ramazan[13] in India, several Hindu organisations across the country organize Iftar parties[14] for Muslim devotees every year. For instance, during Ramazan in 2018, the Mankameshwar Temple in Lucknow organized an Iftar party for the Muslim devotees. Amit Verma writes: "Temple priests, clad in saffron, welcomed Muslim guests and served food after the prayers. . . . The temple committee had made separate arrangements for men and women and what was important was the presence of several leading Muslim clerics at the event" (2018: 15). But the media and the political institutions in India consistently make an effort to erase these narratives of communal collaborations from the daily verbal discussions, from the historical archives, from the media reports, from the libraries, from the institutional curriculums, and ultimately from the memories in order to promote and normalise their fictional narratives of Islamophobia.

Therefore, in order to overcome the habitual practices of Hindu fanaticism and Islamophobia during and after the pandemic of COVID-19, it is important to revive and bring forth these practices of social, cultural, and religious collaborations as a part of habitual existence in contemporary India.

Conclusion

Altogether, this chapter, through identifying and positioning the systemic and epistemic practices of Islamophobia within and outside the parameters of cor-onalogy in contemporary India, has made an effort to generate widely two forms of existential practices that promote non-Islamophobic, de-hierarchical, and socio-culturally inclusive thoughts and actions. They are non-synchronous syn-chronicities and para-modernity. Aditya Nigam understands non-synchronous synchronicities as "life forms and modes of being consigned to the past"' (2020: 29) and para-modernity as a domain that includes those who have been "ban-ished and excluded by the rational secular moderns" (2020: 32). The practices of Islamophobia in the form of killing Muslims for consuming beef, through creat-ing anti-Muslim rumours, through vandalising Muslim religious sites, through criminalising Islamic socio-religious practices, etc., which have been discussed in this chapter show the various ways through which the Muslims in India are being uprooted from their socio-historical past, on the one side, and are expelled from the socio-cultural mainframe, on the other. Therefore, in order to build a non-Islamophobic society in India during and after the COVID-19 pandemic, it is not only important to revive the collaborative and co-creative socio-historical past but to embrace the "different modes of being that constitute the epistemically dispos-sessed" (Nigam, 2020: 38).

Notes

1 The problem of an infodemic, especially during the COVID-19 lockdown in India, is a bigger problem than the ongoing COVID-19 pandemic. Through using the coronavirus pandemic as a weapon, verbal rumours, false articles, and fake videos have been playing an instrumental role in creating Islamophobia across the country.
2 The Dawoodi Bohras are a religious denomination that belongs to the Ismaili branch of Shia Islam.
3 A Hindu religious festival that celebrates the birth of the Hindu god Rama.
4 According to Islam, *Urs* refers to the death anniversary of a Sufi saint, and it is held at the saint's *dargah* (shrine or grave of a reputed Muslim religious figure). Usually this ritual is followed by the Muslims in South Asia.
5 The temple that belongs to the Hindu god Lord Jagannatha.

6 A majority of the Muslim settlers in Assam are immigrants (legal as well as illegal) from Bangladesh. Therefore, generally, the Muslim residents in Assam are identified as foreigners.

7 In the Marathi language, the word *landiya* is used in a derogatory manner and it means "circumcised penises."

8 A term that is used to identify the pastoral community from the lower Indus valley of Sindh.

9 Vishwa Hindu Parishad is an Indian right-wing Hindu social, cultural, and political organisation.

10 The ritualistic prayers offered by the believers/worshippers in Islam.

11 Laziness and disinterest towards gaining and sharing genuine information and knowledge provoke individuals to lethargically rely on rumors and fake news, as has been seen in case of Islamophobic attacks during COVID-19 in India.

12 A Hindu temple that belongs to Lord Shiva.

13 The ninth month of the Islamic calendar.

14 During the month of Ramazan, in order to break their daily fast, the Muslims organise a daily community gathering at sunset. In the gathering, besides offering prayers, they also consume varieties of snacks, sweet items, and fruit juices. This community gathering is referred to as the Iftar party.

References

Akbar, M. J. 1988. *Riot After Riot: Reports on Caste and Communal Violence in India*. New Delhi: Penguin Books.

Ali, W., Clifton, E., Duss, M., Fang, L., Keyes, S. and Shakir, F. 2011. Fear, Inc. The roots of the Islamophobia in North America. *Center for American Progress*, 26 August. www.americanprogress.org/issues/religion/reports/2011/08/26/10165/fear-inc/ (accessed 16 September 2020).

Banerji, R. 2019. From India to China, the world's Muslims are being put into concentration camps. *Independent,* 11 September. www.independent.co.uk/voices/india-bjp-narendra-modi-muslim-detention-camps-assam-bangladesh-a9100886.html (accessed 18 September 2020).

Bazian, H. 2018. Islamophobia, "Clash of civilizations", and forging a post-cold war order! *Religions*, 9(282): 1–13.

BBC News. 2013. Muzaffarnagar: Tales of death and despair in India's riot-hit town. *BBC News*, 25 September. www.bbc.com/news/world-asia-india-24172537 (accessed 17 September 2020).

BBC News. 2017. Muslims on India train assaulted 'because they ate beef'. *BBC*, 24 June. www.bbc.com/news/world-asia-india-40393331 (accessed 20 September 2020).

BBC News. 2020. 1964: Riots in Calcutta leave more than 100 dead. *BBC*, 13 January. http://news.bbc.co.uk/onthisday/hi/dates/stories/january/13/newsid_4098000/4098363.stm#:~:text=Site%20%7C%20Text%20Only-1964%3A%20Riots%20in%20Calcutta%20leave%20more%20than%20100%20dead,spread%20to%20the%20surrounding%20districts (accessed 17 September 2020).

Beaty, K. 2018. Taj Mahal vandalized as Hindu nationalists dispute site's Muslim origins. *Religion News Service*, 19 June. https://religionnews.com/2018/06/19/taj-mahal-vandalized-as-hindu-nationalists-dispute-sites-muslim-origins/ (accessed 19 September 2020).

Bennet, J. 2017. India's cattle traders fear ruin, vigilante attacks following slaughter ban. *ABC News*, 7 June. www.abc.net.au/news/2017-06-07/india-cattle-traders-fear-ruin-vigilante-attacks-slaughter-ban/8595806 (accessed 20 September 2020).

Biswas, S. 2018. Is India waging a 'war' on Islamic names? *BBC*, 13 November. www.bbc.com/news/world-asia-india-46191239 (accessed 18 September 2020).

Chattopadhyay, A. 2020. Fact check: Fake videos shared to defame muslim community for spreading coronavirus. *The Logical Indian*, 2 April. https://thelogicalindian.com/fact-check/muslim-lick-plates-coronavirus-covid-19-pandemic-20429 (accessed 15 September 2020).

Choudhary, R. 2019. Nellie massacre and 'citizenship': When 1,800 Muslims were killed in Assam in just 6 hours. *The Print*, 18 February. https://theprint.in/india/governance/nellie-massacre-and-citizenship-when-1800-muslims-were-killed-in-assam-in-just-6-hours/193694/ (accessed 17 September 2020).

Dawn. 2020. Muslim man in India attacked with hammer on suspicion of transporting beef: media. *Dawn*, 2 August. www.dawn.com/news/1572347 (accessed 20 September 2020).

Desai, S. and Amarasingam, A. 2020. *#CoronaJihad: COVID-19, Misinformation, and Anti-Muslim Violence in India*. London: ISD Global.

Dey, S. 2020. Corona-logy: A re-configuration of racial dynamics in contemporary India. *Mizoram University Journal of Humanities and Social Sciences*, 6(2): 46–58.

Dilshad, M. 2018. For 26 yrs, Muslims have taken care of this temple. *The Times of India*, 17 September. https://timesofindia.indiatimes.com/india/for-26-yrs-muslims-have-taken-care-of-this-temple/articleshow/65835062.cms (accessed 24 September 2020).

Dogra, B. 2016. When Muslim rulers helped and protected hindu temples. *Mainstream Weakly*, 28 November. www.mainstreamweekly.net/article6858.html (accessed 24 September 2020).

Dogra, B. 2019. Recalling the Muslim rulers who built temples. *The New Leam*, 15 January. www.thenewleam.com/2019/01/recalling-the-muslim-rulers-who-built-temples/ (accessed 24 September 2020).

DW. 2017. Muslim man beaten to death over cows in India. *DW*, 5 April. www.dw.com/en/muslim-man-beaten-to-death-over-cows-in-india/a-38301870 (accessed 20 September 2020).

Ernst, C. 2003. *Following Mohammad: Rethinking Islam in the Contemporary World*. Chapel Hill: The University of North Carolina Press.

ET Online. 2019. Citizenship (Amendment) Act 2019: What is it and why is seen as a problem. *The Economic Times*, 31 December. https://economictimes.indiatimes.com/news/et-explains/citizenship-amendment-bill-what-does-it-do-and-why-is-it-seen-as-a-problem/articleshow/72436995.cms?from=mdr (accessed 18 September 2020).

Explained Desk. 2020. Explained: Sections 269 & 270 IPC, invoked against those accused of spreading disease? *The Indian Express*, 30 March. https://indianexpress.com/article/explained/explained-what-are-sections-269-270-ipc-invoked-against-those-accused-of-spreading-disease-6336810/ (accessed 24 May 2023).

Ghosh, P. 2020. Tablighi jamaat congregation: BJP MP it was planned 'corona jihad'. *India.com*, 4 April. www.india.com/news/india/tablighi-jamaat-congregation-bjp-mp-says-it-was-planned-corona-jihad-3990592/ (accessed 14 September 2020).

Grosfoguel, R. 2008. Epistemic islamophobia and colonial social sciences. *Human Architecture: Journal of the Sociology of Self-Knowledge*, 8(2): 29–38.

Haider, T. 2020. Timeline of how Nizamuddin Markaz defied lockdown with 3400 people at Tablighi Jamaat event. *India Today*, 31 March. www.indiatoday.in/india/story/timeline-of-nizamuddin-markaz-event-of-tablighi-jamaat-in-delhi-1661726-2020-03-31 (accessed 14 September 2020).

HT Correspondent. 2014. Hate speech leaders get away with spewing venom. *Hindustan Times*, 21 April. www.hindustantimes.com/india/hate-speech-leaders-get-away-with-spewing-venom/story-c7Eya6JlUmTmjDhQTNelaP.html (accessed 18 September 2020).

Human Rights Watch. 2017. India: 'Cow protection' spurs vigilante violence. *Human Rights Watch*, 27 April. www.hrw.org/news/2017/04/27/india-cow-protection-spurs-vigilante-violence (accessed 20 September 2020).

Human Rights Watch. 2019. India: Citizenship bill discriminates against Muslims. *Human Rights Watch*, 11 December. www.hrw.org/news/2019/12/11/india-citizenship-bill-discriminates-against-muslims (accessed 18 September 2020).

Hussain, T. 2020. 'How is it human?': India's largest detention centre almost ready. *Al Jazeera*, 2 January. www.aljazeera.com/news/2020/01/human-india-largest-detention-centre-ready-200102044649934.html (accessed 18 September 2020).

IANS. 2019. India: For centuries, this Muslim family has been taking care of a Shiva temple in Assam. *Gulf News*, 28 October. https://gulfnews.com/world/asia/india/india-for-centuries-this-muslim-family-has-been-taking-care-of-a-shiva-temple-in-assam-1.1572274462878 (accessed 24 September 2020).

Imam, S. and Salim, S. 2017. Remembering 1980 Moradabad Muslim massacre: A harsh indictment of 'secular' and Left politics. *Firstpost*, 27 June. www.firstpost.com/india/remembering-1980-moradabad-muslim-massacre-a-harsh-indictment-of-lefts-secular-politics-3745717.html (accessed 17 September 2020).

Kapoor, C. 1984. Fury of communal violence burns 80 km stretch from tip of south Bombay to Bhiwandi town. *India Today*, 15 June. www.indiatoday.in/magazine/indiascope/story/19840615-fury-of-communal-violence-burns-80-km-stretch-from-tip-of-south-bombay-to-bhiwandi-town-803038-1984-06-15 (accessed 17 September 2020).

Karmakar, R. 2020. 30 'foreigners' dead in Assam's detention centres. *The Hindu*, 12 April. www.thehindu.com/news/national/30-foreigners-dead-in-assams-detention-centres/article31325045.ece (accessed 18 September 2020).

Kimura, M. 2013. *The Nellie Massacre of 1983: Agency of Rioters*. New Delhi: Sage Publishers.

Krishnan, M. 2020. Indian Muslims face renewed stigma amid COVID-19 crisis. *DW*, 14 May. www.dw.com/en/indian-muslims-face-renewed-stigma-amid-covid-19-crisis/a-53436462 (accessed 15 September 2020).

Mander, H. 2017. Why the Hashimpura massacre of 42 Muslim men in 1987 is relevant in the polarised UP of today. *Scroll.in*, 16 April. https://scroll.in/article/833915/why-the-hashimpura-massacre-of-42-muslim-men-in-1987-is-relevant-in-the-polarised-up-of-today (accessed 17 September 2020).

Matharu, H. 2019. Divide and ruLE: 'Colonial mindsets are fuelling islamophobia and racism. *Byline Times*, 2 July. https://bylinetimes.com/2019/07/02/divide-and-rule-colonial-mindsets-are-fuelling-islamophobia-and-racism/ (accessed 17 September 2020).

Ndlovu-Gatsheni, S. J. 2020. *Decolonization, Decoloniality, and the Future of African Studies: A Conversation with Dr. Sabelo J. Ndlovu-Gatsheni. Interviewed by Duncan Omanga. Items: Insights from the Social Sciences*, 14 January. https://items.ssrc.org/from-our-programs/decolonization-decoloniality-and-the-future-of-african-studies-a-conversation-with-dr-sabelo-ndlovu-gatsheni/ (accessed 14 September 2020).

Niazi, S. 2019. India: Muslim attacked for allegedly selling beef. *Anadolu Agency*, 9 April. www.aa.com.tr/en/asia-pacific/india-muslim-attacked-for-allegedly-selling-beef/1446178# (accessed 20 September 2020).

Nigam, A. 2020. *Decolonizing Theory: Thinking Across Traditions*. New Delhi: Bloomsbury.

Pillalamarri, A. 2019. The origins of Hindu-Muslim conflict in South Asia. *The Diplomat*, 16 March. https://thediplomat.com/2019/03/the-origins-of-hindu-muslim-conflict-in-south-asia/ (accessed 17 September 2020).

Pradhan, B. 2020. Millions in India could end up in modi's new detention camps. *Bloomberg*, 26 February. www.bloomberg.com/features/2020-modi-india-detention-camps/ (accessed 18 September 2020).

Press Trust of India. 2020. Mosque, dargah vandalised in northeast Delhi during violence, claims locals. *India Today*, 27 February. www.indiatoday.in/india/story/delhi-violence-mosque-dargah-vandalised-ashok-nagar-chand-bagh-1650491-2020-02-27 (accessed 19 September 2020).

PTI. 2018. 3 villages in Rajasthan renamed, says MHA – Check list here. *Financial Express*, 9 August. www.financialexpress.com/india-news/3-villages-in-rajasthan-renamed-says-mha-check-list-here/1275625/ (accessed 18 September 2020).

Rahman, S. A. 2020. Coronavirus rumors spark communal violence in India. *VOA News*, 8 July. www.voanews.com/covid-19-pandemic/coronavirus-rumors-spark-communal-violence-india (accessed 15 September 2020).

Regan, H., Sur, P. and Sud, V. 2020. India's Muslims feel targeted by rumors they're spreading COVID-19. *CNN*, 24 April. https://edition.cnn.com/2020/04/23/asia/india-coronavirus-muslim-targeted-intl-hnk/index.html (accessed 15 September 2020).

Safi, M. 2018. Indians 'cow protectors' jailed for life over murder of Muslim man. *The Guardian*, 22 March. www.theguardian.com/world/2018/mar/22/indian-cow-vigilantes-jailed-for-life-alimuddin-ansari-death (accessed 20 September 2020).

Salim, S. 2020. Gujarat Riots – 1969: When congress government helped an anti-Muslim Massacre. *Heritage Times*, 20 January. http://heritagetimes.in/gujarat-riots-congress-1969/ (accessed 17 September 2020).

Samuel, S. 2019. India's massive, scary new detention camps, explained. *Vox*, 17 September. www.vox.com/future-perfect/2019/9/17/20861427/india-assam-citizenship-muslim-detention-camps (accessed 18 September 2020).

Santos, B. D. S. 2016. *Epistemologies of the South: Justice against Epistemicide*. London and New York: Routledge.

Sayyid, S. 2014. A measure of islamophobia. *Islamophobia Studies Journal*, 2(1): 10–25.

Sheehi, S. 2011. *Islamophobia: The Ideological Campaign against Muslims*. Atlanta: Clarity Press.

Siddique, N. 2020. Inside Assam's detention camps: How the Current citizenship crisis disenfranchises Indians. *EPW*, 15 February. www.epw.in/engage/article/inside-assams-detention-camps-how-current (accessed 18 September 2020).

Singh, T. S. 2017. How British Raj's 'divide & rule' policy is still in use by our politicians to remain in power. *The Logical Indian*, 10 October. https://thelogicalindian.com/story-feed/awareness/british-raj-divide-rule-policy/ (accessed 17 September 2020).

Staff Reporter. 2018. Mosque vandalized in Haryana's Karnal. *The Hindu*, 1 June. www.thehindu.com/news/national/other-states/mosque-vandalised-in-haryanas-karnal/article24054933.ece (accessed 19 September 2020).

Tasci, U. N. 2020. The Hindu temples built by Muslims in pre-colonial India. *TRT World*, 12 August. www.trtworld.com/magazine/the-hindu-temples-built-by-muslims-in-pre-colonial-india-38845 (accessed 24 September 2020).

Thompson, P., Itaoui, R. and Bazian, H. 2019. *Islamophobia in India: Stoking Bigotry*. Berkeley: Islamophobia Studies Center.

Trivedi, S. 2020. Coronavirus: The story of India's largest COVID-19 cluster. *The Hindu*, 11 April. www.thehindu.com/news/national/coronavirus-nizamuddin-tablighi-jamaat-markaz-the-story-of-indias-largest-covid-19-cluster/article31313698.ece (accessed 14 September 2020).

Verma, A. 2018. Ancient Hindu temple in Uttar Pradesh hosts iftar party for Muslims. *Deccan Chronicle*, 12 June. www.deccanchronicle.com/nation/current-affairs/120618/ancient-hindu-uttar-pradesh-temple-hosts-iftar-party-for-muslims.html (accessed 24 September 2020).

Vetticad, A. M. 2020. India media accused of Islamophobia for its coronavirus coverage. *Al Jazeera*, 15 May. www.aljazeera.com/news/2020/04/indian-media-accused-islamophobia-coronavirus-coverage-200417064109353.html (accessed 15 September 2020).

INDEX

Access to COVID-19 Tools (ACT)
        Accelerator 50
actualisation, ontology of 30
Addams, Jane 29
aesthetic ethics 33
Africa/African: labour 111;
        public health 133
African Union (AU) 43, 52, 66;
        Agenda 2063 54
aggression 5, 30
Akbar, M.J. 146
Alexander, J. 31
Allen, V. L. 116
Amarasingam, A. 142
Amnesty International 80–81
Anderson, J. 43, 44
Anglo Platinum Khuseleka Mine
        116–117, 122
Ansari, A. 152
anti-migration 47
anti-Muslims 145, 150
apartheid laws 118
Appadurai, A. 32, 48, 49
Archaeological Survey of India (ASI) 151
Armstrong, D. 63
artificial intelligence (AI) 97
ASI see Archaeological Survey of India (ASI)
Assam 147, 149, 150, 152, 154
Association of Mineworkers and
        Construction Union (AMCU) 115,
        116, 118
asylum seekers 52–53

AU see African Union (AU)
authoritarian/authoritarianism 5, 30;
        governments 14; leadership 32;
        regimes 13, 14; turn 78; use of 29

Babri Masjid (Babri Mosque) 151
Bachelet, M. 79
"bad-human" behaviour 100
Barraud YouTube channel 133, 134
Barry, B. 45
Bazian, H. 150
Bennet, J. 152
Bharatiya Janta Party (BJP) 142, 148, 150
Bhatt, E. 32
Bhiwandi riots in 1984 147
Bhopal chemical disaster in India 119
Bieber, F. 45–46
BJP see Bharatiya Janta Party (BJP)
Black Africans 3–4
Black labourers 92
Black Lives Matter (BLM) protests 100
Black mineworkers 6, 109, 111, 112, 118,
        121–122; at Anglo Platinum 118;
        compensation for 110–111; housing
        conditions of 122
blaming, patterns of 144
Blaut, J.M. 44, 45
BLM protests see Black Lives Matter (BLM)
        protests
Boko Haram attacks 69
Bosancianu, C. M. 13
Botswana 51–52, 111, 118, 121, 122

brand Islamophobia 150
bubonic plague 92, 143
bureaucracy 43
Butler, J. 31, 32
Buzan, B. 96, 101

Cambridge Analytica scandal 94–95
Campbell, J. 69
Canada 10; delivery of public goods in
    14–19; interventions in 19–20;
    outbreak in 14; persons and
    monetary values in 15–17; vaccines 4
capitalism 3, 102, 103; data 98–102; for
    economic benefit 92; racial 98–102
Capoccia, G. 46, 51
cathedral thinking 31
Center for Policy Research in
    New Delhi 143
Chamberlain, W. 50
Chantal, M. 34
Chernobyl nuclear disaster 119
China/Chinese 2, 4, 14, 30; COVID-19
    vaccines 4; virus *see* coronavirus;
    Wuhan lockdown in 31
Cilliers, J. 98
civic nationalism 46–48, 54
civilisation 30, 35, 43, 142
civil society 101–102, 130
claimants, categories of 119
climate change, challenges of 31
closed-circuit television (CCTV)
    cameras 95–96
Colijn, C. 50–51, 53
co-living 29
collaborative/collaboration 154; communal
    154–155; leadership 32;
    self-organisation 32–33; well-being
    33–34
colonialism 3, 6, 102; exploration of
    95; forms of 94; historical 97;
    traditional forms of 93, 97
coloniality 6, 103, 114, 118, 124
colonial superpowers 6, 104
colonisation 93–94, 97, 104
Commission of Inquiry into Mine Safety
    and Health 111
communal collaborations 154–155
communal hate 150
communal scapegoating, culture of 143
compensation 112; claims for 122;
    process of 120
conceptualisation 43–46; nation,
    nationalism, and nationalisms 43–46

Congolese diaspora 6, 128, 129, 131,
    132–134
Congolese migrants 128, 131–132, 134, 136
Connolly, W. 32
constitutive violence 35
constructivism 31
contact tracing 67, 96, 97, 131, 144
containment, public policies of 30
contemporary human civilisation 30
cordon sanitaire 63
#CoronaJihad 141–145; Bhiwandi riots in
    1984 147; brand Islamophobia 150;
    gastronomic Islamophobia
    151–152; geographical
    Islamophobia 150–151; Gujarat
    riots of 1969 146; Hashimpura
    massacre in 1987 147–148;
    Hindu-centric Islamophobia
    145; Kolkata riots in 1964 146;
    Moradabad riots in 1980 146–147;
    Muzaffarpur riots in 2013 148–150;
    Nellie massacre in 1983 147;
    RDC (realisation-depolarisation-
    collaboration) model 152–155
corona nationalism 49
coronationalism, notion of 49–50
coronavirus: crisis, critical genealogy and
    ontology of 30; emergence of 1
Couldry, N. 93, 97, 99
COVID-19: before and after 1; alternative
    planetary futures 35–36; colonialism
    2; consequences of 79–80; context
    of 9; death and destruction 29;
    diplomacy 14; disproportionate
    effects of 4–5, 9; economic impacts
    of 12–13; ethical issues 33; global
    financial crisis of 2008–2009 2;
    and global health 10–12; infections
    120; interventions to businesses
    18–19; issues and impacts of 4; link
    between data and 95–97; literature
    on 9; lockdowns 5; misinformation
    and myths about 128; moment,
    description of 42–43; narrow
    nationalism in Southern Africa
    51–53; nationalism and sub-forms
    49–51; national response to 128;
    planetary impacts of 2–3; political
    impacts of response to 13–14;
    precautionary social controls 12;
    prevention messages in public
    places 136; protocols 122; public
    health responses to 13; reality

and existence of 135; recognising 10–11; rules and regulations 5; social impacts of responses to 12; on social services 69; spiritual calling of 33–35; state responses to 14–24; vaccine trials 135
COVID-19 Tools (ACT) Accelerator 19–20
COVID-19 Vaccines Global Access Facility (COVAX) 19–20, 50
creative leadership 32
crimes against humanity 76, 132
criminalisation 149
Critchley, S. 34
critical junctures 51
cultivate immortality 35
cultural diversity 32
culturecides 142
cyberspace 97–99; nature of 98

Das, V. 30, 33
data capitalism 98–102
data colonialism 6, 93–94, 98, 102, 103; during COVID-19 pandemic in South Africa 94–95; definition of 90–91
data mining companies 94–95
Davenport, C. 98
Dawoodi Bohra community 143
death-bound subjectivity 114
deaths 12–14, 32, 34, 64–66, 109, 111–116
deborderisation, challenges of 32–33
decolonisation 3, 6, 124
democracy, reputation of 14
Democratic Republic of the Congo (DRC) 6, 127–128, 135; Congolese migrants and public response to COVID-19 pandemic in 131–136; transnationalism and public health governance in 128
Department of Justice Canada 14
depolarisation 153–154
Desai, S. 142
detention centres 151
digital space 98–99, 102, 103–104
Disaster Management Act 57 of 2002 of South Africa 93, 96
disciplinary nationalism 50
discrimination 146, 149
DRC see Democratic Republic of the Congo (DRC)

Ebola 66, 78, 131, 132
economic/economy: hardships 131; impact payments 21; inequalities 6, 102; recovery 21
education, institutions of 2
Eid 146
emotional imbalances 129
endemic poverty 29
entanglement 61
environmental destruction 123
environmental pollution 129
epidemic of ignorance 30
epistemicides 142
epistemic violence 145
epistemological Islamophobia 152
Ernst, J. 114
Escobar, A. 32
ethnic cleansing 76
ethnicity 100
ethnic nationalism 46–47
Euro-American–based Congolese migrants 129
European scientific community 3

Facebook 95, 133, 134
facial recognition 98, 99–100
Faleye, O. A. 62
false criminal charges 150
Fang, F. 31
Fanon, G. 114
fatalism 30, 31
February riots in Delhi 143
Felson, M. 67
Floyd, G. 29
Food and Agricultural Organization (FAO) 66
food security 55, 62, 66, 67
Foucault, M. 30
Fukushima nuclear disaster 119

Ganguly, M. 149, 152
gastronomic Islamophobia 151–152
Gates, M. 3
Gemma, B. 61
geographical Islamophobia 150–151
Gibson-Fall, F. 78
Gilhooly, M. 114
Global Affairs Canada 19–20
global health history 62
globalisation 2, 42; assaults the values of 5
global North 2–3
global political economy 4, 9
global responsibility 31

global security 61–62
global South 2–4
global virus morbidity 61
glocal insurgency 63
Gordon, L. R. 114
GoS *see* government of South Africa (GoS)
government of South Africa (GoS) 76;
     commitment to R2P 82; Disaster
     Management Act 80; Emergency
     Services Act 76; National Health
     Act 76; personal protective
     equipment (PPE) distribution 80
Greer, S. L. 13
guinea pigs 6, 134, 136
Gujarat riots of 1969 146

Habermas, J. 30
Haraway, D. 32
Hashimpura massacre in 1987 147–148
Haushofer, J. 11
health: care system 20; governance
     6, 73, 128–129; security 63;
     transnationalism 128–130, 136
hegemonic order 123
He, Q. 13
Hindu: anti-Islamic practices 150; fanaticism
     150; fanatics 141, 142; Islamophobia
     145, 149; and Muslim harmony
     154; and Muslim riot 146–147
historical colonialism 97
historical institutionalism 46
Hofman, K. 82
Honneth, A. 35
Horton, R. 34
human entanglements 5, 42, 43
human health 1, 4, 62
humanitarian responsibilities, forms of 142
humanity 2, 42, 46, 56
human life 12, 35
human mobility 63, 127
human rights 111; protection 77–79;
     realisation 83–85; violations 2, 80–81
Human Rights Watch 149
hunger 53, 114, 135

Ibrahim, S. 151
imagined communities 43–45
Imam, S. 147
imperialism 3
Independent Investigative Policy Directorate
     (IPID) 81
India 145; Citizenship Amendment
     Bill (CAB) 149; community

in 149–150; divide and rule
     framework 148; divisive tendencies
     in 7; Islamophobic practices in
     145; lockdown in 35; political
     institutions in 154–155
indigenous remedies 132, 135, 136
individualism 33
industrial disasters 119
inequality 5–7, 25, 69, 93, 95, 100, 102
information communication and
     technologies (ICTs) 130, 132–133
intercontinental citizenship 129
International Labour Organisation
     (ILO) 112
international migration studies 129
International Organisation for Migration
     (IOM) 68
international relations 43, 60
IPID *see* Independent Investigative Policy
     Directorate (IPID)
Islamic existence, systemic and epistemic
     erasure of 149–150
Islamophobia: brand 150; in contemporary
     India 145; epistemological and
     ontological frameworks of 145,
     148; fictional narratives of 155;
     gastronomic 151–152; geographical
     150–151; Hindu-centric 145
Islamophobia in India: Stoking Bigotry
     (Thompson, Itaoui, and Hatem) 150
Islamophobic narratives 141, 142
Itaoui, R. 150

Jaina tradition 34
Jallianwala Bagh 147
Jamaat, T. 153
Jan-Mohamed, A. 114
Jeeves, A. H. 116
Jowitt, S. M. 122
Justice for Miners Campaign (J4C) group
     119–120

Kane, J. 44
Karandlaje, S. 142
Kelemen, R. D. 46, 51
Kendall-Taylor, A. 14
Khuseleka mine 109
Kimura, M. 147
King Jr., M. L. 33–34
knowledge: of nature and culture 61–62;
     production matrix 55
Kolkata riots in 1964 146
kongo-bololo 132, 137

labour: activities, virtual space for 6;
    intellectual division of 3; markets,
    vulnerable segments of 6; traditional
    viewpoint of 99
Laclau, E. 34
Lamberk, M. 33
latent nationalism 45–46
Latour, B. 30
law enforcement: agencies 98–99; practical
    application of 100
leadership: collaborative/collaboration 32;
    creative 32; ethics and responsibility 81
leapfrogging, concept of 98
learning, institutions of 2
Lemba, L. N. 135
Leon Commission of Inquiry in 1994 113
Lesotho 110, 121, 122
Lever, A. 99–100
linguicides 142
lockdown 2, 35, 51–53, 65, 120, 122;
    enforcement 78, 81, 83–85;
    environment 79; implementation
    of 11; in India 35; measures 77,
    80–81; procedures 42; short-term
    52; strategy 52
Longondo, E. 135–136

Madhi, S. 82
Magubane, B. 110, 115–116, 118
Magufuli, J. P. 133
Makhanya, S. 116, 118
Maldonado-Torres, N. 115–116
Mandela, N. 111
market orientation 10
mass inequality 95
mass testing for COVID-19 131
Mbatha, M. W. 67
Mbeki, T. 123
Mbemba, T. 135
Mbembe, A. 29, 35
McCulloch, J. 117
mediation, process of 114
Medical Bureau for Occupational Diseases
    (MBOD) 112
medical facilities 136
medical nationalism 49
Meel, B. 110, 117
Mejias, U. A. 93, 97, 99
mental trauma 114–115
mental well-being 130
Metcalf, C. J. E. 11
migrants/migration 2, 128, 130; literature
    131–132; networks 129–130;
    transnationalism among 132–133

miners, compensation for 110
Miners' Phthisis Allowance Act (Act No. 34
    of 1911) 110
mineworkers 118, 120; compensating 122;
    health of 114–115; housing for 115;
    ill-health of 118; killers of 116; in
    social violence 114–115; in South
    Africa 110
mining: companies 119; industry 112,
    116, 121; management, syndicate
    inclusive of 118
modernity 34
Moodie, T. D. 123
Moradabad riots in 1980 146–147
mortality 13, 26, 34, 35
Motsoaledi, A. 113
movement restrictions 63, 66
Moyo, Z. 50, 52, 56
Mozambique 51, 110
Mukumbang, F. C. 52
Mulkay, M. 114
multi-dimensional transformations 36
multi-faith, India 154
multi-temporal hermeneutics 33
Munyangi, Jerome 135
Muslims 141; community 154; during
    COVID-19 145; discrimination of
    149; economic existence of 153;
    in India 153; marginalization and
    exclusion of 145; owned buildings
    146; physical violence against 148;
    socio-economic existence of 151;
    vandalization of 151
mutual organisation 32–33
Muyembe, J.-J. 134, 135
Muzaffarpur riots in 2013 148–150

Namibia 51–52
Narayan, H. 13, 147
narratives of distractions 144
narrow nationalism 44–45, 49, 53, 56;
    human entanglements and solutions
    to 53–56
Naseerudin, H. M. 143
National Corona Virus Command Councill
    (NCCC) 75
nationalism 53–54; concept of 44; forms of
    43, 46–50; history of 44; narrow
    application of 46; for real-world
    nationalists 45; revolutionary and
    progressive force of 46; tendencies
    of exclusion 47; toxic side of 48
national lockdowns 2
National Mineworkers union (NUM) 112

National Policy on Food and Nutritional
    Security 67
national sovereignty 49
nation-state borders 127
Ndhlovu, F. 44
Ndlovu-Gatsheni, S. J. 44
Nellie massacre in 1983 147
neo-capitalism 99
neoliberalism 10, 25
neoliberal state 9
Nigam, A. 152
Nigeria, lockdowns in 66
non-governmental organisations
    (NGOs) 119
non-Islamic socio-cultural gatherings 144
non-Islamophobic society 153
non-pharmaceutical interventions
    (NPIs) 11
normality 36
Nussbaum, M. 33

Occupational Diseases in Mines and Works,
    Act No. 78 of 1973 (ODMWA)
    111–113
occupational health in mining industry
    109–110; Black mineworker 122–
    123; condemned to death 116–118;
    lung diseases 110; post-COVID
    mining order 121–122; silicosis
    see silicosis; social death in zone of
    non-being 114–115
official nationalisms 43–44
ontological Islamophobia 152
ontological market orientation 10
ontological violence 145
oppression, forms of 102
overcrowding 123

paid compensation 113
pathogenic transmission 65
patriotism 49
personal protective equipment (PPE)
    20, 121
physical Islamophobia 152
physical violence, against Muslims 148
physical well-being 130
pneumonia 127
police brutality 101
political leaders 54
political/politics: economy, decolonisation
    of 6; identity 47; ideology 44–45;
    transformations 32, 33
political turmoil 131
poverty 3, 5, 25, 111, 117, 122, 131

power 9–10, 65; consolidation and
    centralisation of 78–79; COVID-19
    see COVID-19; distribution
    63; global frame of power 65;
    institutions and structures of 142;
    knowledge and 95; networks of
    mobile culture 67–68; spatialisation
    of 62–63, 68; of state for public
    goods 25; systemic exchange of 93
preferentiality, reality of 62
prejudice 36, 101
Prevention of Cruelty to Animal Act on 26
    May_2017 151
psychological imbalances 129
psychological trauma 114–115
public goods, power of state for 25
public health 21; African 133; biopolitics
    and geopolitics of 60; crisis
    10–11; governance 128–131;
    instrumentality of 69; interventions
    67; measures 70; policies 65–66;
    promotion 82; sector 129

quarantine centres 132, 136

R2P see responsibility to protect (R2P)
race/racial/racism 5, 29, 100; capitalism
    98–102; inequality, hierarchical
    nature of 100; injustices 110–111;
    policies, legacy of 25; profiling 98,
    99–100; segregation 100–101
radical dehumanization 34
radicalisation 69
Rahman, H. M. 154
Rajagopal, P.V. 32
Rajoelina, A. 133
Ramazan 154
rationality 33, 154
RDC (realisation-depolarisation-
    collaboration) model 152–155
realisation 153
Reardon, J. 31
reconfiguration, process of 142
Rees, D. 121, 122
regional reality 70
regional stability 60
religious beliefs 154
religious traditions 34
repercussions 5
responsibility: challenges of 30–31; visions
    and practices of 31
responsibility to protect (R2P) 5, 76–78, 80,
    82, 84, 85; concept 77; principle
    77–79

Rossi, A. 95–96
Rouvinski, V. 14
Roy, A. 36
Russia 4, 14
Rustenburg 109

SADC Health Protocol 130
Salim, S. 146, 147
Samuel, S. 149
San, S. 14
Sayyid, S. 145
scapegoating, history of 143
scepticism 3, 136
Schiller, N. G. 130
scientific knowledge 61
securitisation of borders 2
self-awareness 153
self-investigation 153
self-realisation 153
sense of discrimination 146
Shah, A. 150
Sharma, N. 144
silicosis 109, 120; continued exposure to
    115–116; COVID-19, tuberculosis
    and 120; diagnostic and testing
    centres for 121; history of 109–110;
    landmark 110; prevalence of 116;
    ruling for mineworkers 119–120;
    in South African mines 110–114;
    and TB 115, 117; underlining
    conditions 120; victims of 112
sinister motives 142
Sinopharm 4
Sinovac 4
slave trade 3, 97, 99
slave wage 110
Smith, I. 45
social contract 4–5, 9, 82, 84
social death 114–115; existence/
    non-existence of 114
social distancing 2, 11, 70, 75, 76, 80,
    115, 135
social inequalities 6, 102
social justice in South Africa 91
social media 136, 141; accounts 95;
    platforms 94, 95, 98
social networks 64
social relations 102
social science 56
social security, provision of 67
social segregation 100–101
social stigmatisation 96–97
social trauma 110

society: socio-cultural fabric of 12; spatial
    pattern of 61
socio-economic inequalities 7
socio-economic remittances 130
solidarity, challenges of 30–31
Sondela 109, 118
South Africa 51–52, 74–76; Black migrant
    workers in 123; colonialism and
    apartheid in 91; colonisations of
    91–92; conceptual dimensions
    76–77; COVID-19 1, 77–80,
    97–98; data: colonialism 91;
    decolonising 102–104; Disaster
    Management Act, 2002 5; divide-
    and-rule strategy 93; history of
    mining in 110–114; human rights:
    abuses during the COVID-19
    lockdown 80–83; litigation
    process 119; mining industry in
    116, 121; National Disaster Act
    101; plagues during colonial
    92–93; platinum mines in 122; post-
    apartheid 93; and racial capitalism
    98–102; realisation and lockdown
    enforcement balance 83–85;
    separateness in 104
South Africa First (SAF) 53
South African Minerals Council 121
South African National Defence Forces
    (SANDF) 80, 82, 101
South African Police Service (SAPS) 80–82
Southern Africa Development Community
    (SADC) 51
Southern Africa, narrow nationalism in
    51–53
Southern African Community
    Development (SADC) region
    110, 129
Southern Africa, rural communities
    111–112
sovereignty 44, 49
spirituality 33–34
Sputnik V 4
statistical discrimination 99–100
Stefan, E. 61
Stickle, B. 67
Stilz, A. 47, 54
structural inequality 5
surveillance mechanisms 100
Sweeting, H. 114

Tabassum, H. 142
Tablighi Jamaat 141, 144, 151

Tamir, Y. 47
technology: of contact 132–133; use of 94
Tharoor, S. 149–150
Thompson, P. 150
Thurnberg, G. 30, 31
Tisdell, C. A. 12
toxic nationalism 48–49, 54
transdisciplinarity 55
transformations: challenges of 32–33; multi-dimensional 32, 36; political 32, 33; struggles for 33–34
transnational health practices 131
transnational infectious disease 64
transnationalism: among migrants 132–133; conceptualisation and theorisation of 129–130; health 128, 129–130; notions of 128; and public health governance in 128; and public health governance 129, 130–131
transportation, infrastructure 64
trauma: challenges of 30–31; construction of 31; of virus 30–31
travel bans 12–13
tribalism 44, 47
Trojan horse: colonialism and apartheid in 91; colonisations of 91–92; data colonialism 93–94; description of 90–91
Trump, D. 1, 48, 52
Tshiamiso Trust Fund 119
Tshisekedi, F. 127–128, 136
tuberculosis (TB) 109, 113, 120, 121

ubuntu, concept 103
UN Convention on Civil and Political Rights 82
unemployment 11
unemployment insurance fund (UIF) 53
UN General Assembly (UNGA) Resolution 76
United Nations Human Rights Commissioner 79
United Nations Sustainable Development Goal 3 (UNSDG-3) 77

UN Office for West Africa and the Sahel (UNOWAS) 69
unofficial colonisation 92
UN World Summit 2005 76
urban migration 122
USA 10, 25; businesses and monetary value in 22–23; delivery of public goods in 20–24; Department of the Treasury 20–21; interventions in 24–25; monetary value in 21, 24

vaccine/vaccinations 3, 20, 24–25, 97, 132; on animals 134; apartheid 50; for COVID-19 121; distribution of 3; nationalism 3–4, 49–50; trials 136
Van Onselen, C. 116
Vattimo, G. 30
victimisation 149
violence 91, 143, 150; constitutive 35; Hindu-centred anti-Muslim 145; through coronavirus 141–142
Vishwa Hindu Parishad (VHP) 151

West Africa 60; conceptual clarifications 61–64; public health in 60; state boundaries in 64; transnational responses and security entanglement in 64–70
Western modernity 123
WhatsApp 95, 133, 134
white miners 116
Wolfers, A. 62
World Health Organization (WHO) 1, 50, 64, 97, 112, 127
Wuhan, COVID-19 pandemic in 64

xenophobia 47

Yan, B. 13
yoga 35
YouTube 133

Zimbabwe 47, 51–52, 54
Zizek, S. 30

For Product Safety Concerns and Information please contact our EU
representative GPSR@taylorandfrancis.com
Taylor & Francis Verlag GmbH, Kaufingerstraße 24, 80331 München, Germany

www.ingramcontent.com/pod-product-compliance
Lightning Source LLC
Chambersburg PA
CBHW060309220326
41598CB00027B/4282

9 781032 540993